Matthew . J

CW00497040

Our Enigma

A father and son learning to decode each other's world.

Copyright Notice

Foreword

When attempting to describe a condition, the use of language can often spark disagreement, especially when addressing a condition that affects a significant number of individuals in various ways. As of completing this book in 2023, if you were to read it twenty years from now, there will likely be terms that evoke discomfort or expressions that have become obsolete.

Even within the few years I've dedicated to writing our story, changes have occurred. One instance is the phrasing when referring to someone with autism like my son Rory– is it 'Does Rory have autism?' or 'Is Rory autistic?' I've predominantly chosen the latter, as it aligns with the preference of much of the autistic community. This approach has consistently steered my writing, aiming to use language that resonates with others, though I acknowledge that it might not universally apply, and for that, I extend my apologies.

Regarding language, this book will alternate between English and American spellings of words. This choice stems from the fact that the book was created using various computing platforms over the years, aiming to serve as a guide for both English-speaking book markets.

In addition, child safeguarding holds immense importance, not just in the present but also for Rory's well-being as an autistic adult in the future. When it comes to memoirs or books involving vulnerable individuals, altering their names should be a fundamental ethical consideration. This practice safeguards Rory's privacy and shields him from potential harm or embarrassment that might stem from exposing the intimate details of his life without his future consent. Furthermore, it recognizes that, as he matures, Rory should have the autonomy to decide whether he wants his past experiences and personal stories to be made public. Modifying the names in a memoir not only respects Rory's current vulnerability but also acknowledges the potential long-term consequences of disclosing sensitive information without his consent, ensuring his dignity and agency remain intact as he navigates into adulthood. To uphold these principles, all names, except for my own, have been altered in this book, and certain dates have also been adjusted to provide added protection for both Rory and other individuals featured in the memoir.

So, what is autism?

Autism Spectrum Disorder (ASD) encompasses a complex set of developmental challenges, characterized by difficulties in social interaction, communication, and the presence of restricted and repetitive behaviour. Typically, parents begin to observe signs of autism within the first two to three years of their child's life, with symptoms often manifesting gradually. While some individuals with autism initially meet developmental milestones at a typical pace, their progress may subsequently deteriorate.

The aetiology of autism is attributed to a combination of genetic and environmental factors. During pregnancy, certain infections such as rubella, as well as exposure to toxins like valproic acid, alcohol, cocaine, pesticides, and air pollution, are identified as potential risk factors. Other environmental causes have sparked controversy, including the now-debunked vaccine hypotheses. The condition affects information processing in the brain by altering the connections and organization of nerve cells and their synapses, although the precise mechanisms remain poorly understood. It is worth noting that autism exists on a spectrum, encompassing milder forms of the condition previously referred to as Asperger syndrome or pervasive developmental disorder not otherwise specified (PDD-NOS). However, these distinctions have now been consolidated under the umbrella term autism spectrum disorder. The autistic

2

community, consisting of both caregivers like me and individuals living with the condition like my son Rory, have expressed a dislike for the term "disorder," which has prompted a gradual shift in terminology towards Autism Spectrum Condition (ASC) which while I do acknowledge here. I'll adhere to using ASD for the book, as this is the most likely abbreviation you'll encounter early on from clinicians throughout your own journey.

When I began researching for this book, autism was estimated to affect approximately 24.8 million individuals globally as of 2015. However, recent estimates now suggest the number has increased significantly, reaching closer to that of 79 million.

Over the years, the prevalence of the condition among children in the United States has also risen substantially. The Centres for Disease Control and Prevention (CDC) reported an increase from 1 in 110 children in 2006 to 1 in 54 in 2016. As of the middle of 2023, the current figure stands at 1 in 36 children.

The diagnosis process typically occurs after age 4, but it is possible to reliably diagnose it as early as age 2. Among children with the condition, 31% have an intellectual disability, 25% fall into the borderline range, and 44% have above-average IQ scores.

Autism affects individuals from all ethnic and socioeconomic backgrounds, although minority groups often receive diagnoses later and less frequently. Early intervention is crucial for promoting healthy development and reaping lifelong benefits, despite the lack of medical detection for the condition.

Associated challenges include a significant number of nonverbal or like Rory, minimally verbal individuals. Nearly half of those with autism are prone to wandering, and bullying affects two-thirds of autistic children aged 6 to 15. Self-injurious behaviours are common, and drowning remains a leading cause of death for wandering children.

Autism can impact various aspects of the body and is frequently accompanied by comorbidity (more than one) condition such as attention deficit hyperactivity disorder (ADHD), chronic sleep problems, anxiety, depression, or even gastrointestinal disorders. Approximately one-third of autistic people also experience epilepsy, while schizophrenia affects a considerable percentage of adults.

Health problems related to the condition often extend from early childhood to senior years, with a significant proportion of 2 to 5-year-olds being overweight or obese. While medications like risperidone, sertraline and aripiprazole are sometimes approved to manage autism-associated agitation and irritability.

The financial burden of the condition is substantial, with an estimated welfare and home life cost of $60,000 / £47,000 per year during childhood. Mothers of autistic or disabled children often face reduced work opportunities and lower earnings compared to mothers of children without health limitations or disabilities.

Notably, autism is more prevalent in boys, occurring four times more frequently than in girls. The number of diagnosed cases has risen exponentially since the 1960s, primarily due to changes in diagnostic practices. However, the question of whether actual prevalence rates have increased remains unresolved.

In essence, the condition presents an intricate and challenging journey for both those born with autism and those who care for them. As someone who has been a parent and carer to my son Rory for over a decade, I am acutely aware of the hurdles those new to the condition face, particularly during the pre- and early post-diagnosis stages. At challenging times I've been frustrated, angry, tired, and driven to tears, as there have been moments when certain activities and life experiences seem nearly impossible to navigate or understand the reasoning for such behaviourally puzzling enigmas.

Contents

Introduction

Disclaimer: Before delving into the narrative, it is essential to acknowledge that this book does not provide a comprehensive guide to parenting a child with autism. Rather, it comprises a collection of personal anecdotes and suggestions from my own experiences or those shared with me by others. It is crucial to recognize that every family with an autistic member is unique, and I do not claim that their experiences mirror mine. Furthermore, it is advisable to approach certain chapter subjects with a sense of humour. The stories shared here are infused with love and affection, and in the face of challenges, it is often preferable to find humour in ourselves and the situations we encounter. Over the years, I have read other literature and scientific papers on the topics discussed in this book. However, it is crucial to note that all the opinions and thoughts expressed herein are my own interpretation and may not always align with the latest scientific research and data.

While I will endeavour to explain autism spectrum disorder (ASD) to those who may be less familiar with it in simple terms, it is crucial to remember that each individual on the spectrum is vastly different from the next, just as I am likely to differ from you, the reader. Yes, we may share some common interests and thoughts, but beyond that, we are unique individuals. The same applies to individuals on the spectrum; they possess their own characters, dreams, aspirations, fears, and intelligence, albeit with certain commonalities associated with their diagnosis.

They say everyone has a story within them, and while that may be true, the challenge lies in determining where to begin and what to write about. For most of us, the easiest approach is to draw from what we know or have personally experienced. In my case, that revolves around my own life and, more specifically, my son Rory, who happens to be autistic. Although I have never aspired to write a great work of fiction akin to "Lord of the Rings" or "Harry Potter," I have recently felt compelled to write about my journey as a bumbling father to a remarkable little boy who also happens to be my son. The idea of writing a book gained further traction after discussing my intentions with Bryan, who is not only my closest friend but the only person I have shared my emotions, concerns, and vulnerabilities with over the years. However, recalling his response and the memories associated with it was not something I particularly wished to relive, let alone share with an unknown audience.

Bryan: "Matty, that sounds really good, and you should include your past mental health struggles and breakdown."

Me: "I wasn't planning to include such personal details." But Bryan interrupted, asserting that my son's well-being and that of my daughter were major contributing factors to my previous mental decline. He believed that Rory's condition and his struggle to express emotions or communicate effectively had ultimately impacted my own state of mind. According to Bryan, I had to incorporate the more taboo subjects of disability, divorce, depression, and even suicide in my account of raising a child who was different. The aim was to demonstrate that others experiencing similar thoughts and actions are not alone. It is no secret that marriages involving one or more disabled children often face significant strain or may even disintegrate due to the pervasive influence of autism on both the affected child and the entire family. Reluctantly, I acquiesced to Bryan's advice, as he was generally correct. Thus, he and my partner, Jennifer, became my go-to sources for guidance on such matters. While I don't always follow their advice to the letter, I often seek it to gain a balanced perspective on my intentions.

Therefore, the purpose of this book is to share what I have learned thus far as a father through my own experiences, trials, and errors, and, most importantly, the cultivation of patience and empathy on both my part and Rory's. It is widely acknowledged that mothers bear the brunt of child-rearing worldwide, as the bond between a mother and child during pregnancy and birth is a force to be reckoned with. They are inseparable as one and the same until the day of birth. But sometimes, as fathers, we forget just how significant our role is in our children's lives as role models, protectors, and providers of entertainment. I have made mistakes in this regard, and I will recount them later as I narrate my story of denial, my initial refusal to accept that my son was different from his peers, the subsequent breakdown I experienced, the loss of a job I once enjoyed, family conflicts, and my eventual separation from my wife and children.

I will share my thoughts during that period when I believed no one could understand Rory, and how his school and the local authorities seemed to give up on him. I will recount how a social services intervention, ultimately, led to Rory coming to live with me and Jen in 2017

I have in the past been described as a "Man's Man" and as embodying other masculine clichés. From an outsider's perspective, I might indeed fit that mold, with my relatively broad, strong physique, just shy of six feet in height, and a bald head. I have always enjoyed contact sports like rugby, karate, and judo. I have had some military experience and worked as a doorman, commonly referred to as a bouncer. I left school with no GCSEs and skipped college entirely. Driven by the prospect of money being the driving force behind life's successes, I've worked in retail, insurance, shipping, security, and the military. I've even had my own gardening maintenance company, a wedding photography and videography business. I've been a postman and more recently, I've been involved in education and the sciences fields.

I really am just your average middle-aged, overweight, and bumbling man, but I came into my own and found more purpose in my life and to any material wealth when I became a father to a unique little boy. So, as the saying goes, you should never judge a book by its cover, and I hope to serve as living proof of that.

Through this book, I aim to honestly share my experiences with depression and suicidal thoughts—the tears I've shed—and the way my children, and in particular Rory, ultimately give my life purpose and more direction.

Most importantly, I want to emphasize to fathers that it is completely normal to feel fear and uncertainty when they have a child who is undeniably unique.

Over a decade on I couldn't be prouder of the progress Rory has made, albeit not as swiftly as his sister or typical peers. The real challenge for those starting out, is that we often don't fully grasp the intelligence and understanding that our children possess until much later in their lives, because they often lack the social communication skills to do so in a conventional (termed neurotypical) manner. I now understand that Rory was listening attentively and absorbs much more than he reveals. He also teaches himself skills that neither his teachers nor we were aware he possessed until he simply demonstrates them seemingly out of nowhere.

While I would classify Rory as moderately to severely affected within several areas of the spectrum, it is challenging to define any child as they develop. Some individuals with the condition excel academically, while others do not. Some are verbal, while others communicate in ways that neurotypical individuals like myself may have struggled to understand. As I mentioned earlier, no two autistic individuals are exactly alike.

As our children develop, they find coping strategies and what might once have been considered atypical for a child such as Rory, like delayed speech at the age of two or three, was merely a temporary delay while his brain processed how to communicate in a manner that I or others could comprehend. I now know that he was communicating with me even before he could speak, although I simply failed to grasp the signs and signals before me.

While Rory does still exhibit some atypical behaviours associated with autism, such as in the past hand flapping or repeated words or phrases (echolalia). Over time, some of those preconceived traits have changed or disappeared. While traits like struggling to maintain eye contact have never been an issue for Rory and have been present throughout and that continues to be the case. So, like any individuals, those on the spectrum or otherwise, Rory is constantly learning and adapting.

Rory is a bright light in my life, filling it with laughter and unconditional love. However, both parents and children have their down days, and this is particularly likely if your own child differs somewhat from their peers physiologically or neurologically. I'm here to say its normal to experience such days, and in this book, I aim to discuss them openly and honestly with you, the reader.

The challenge now lies in determining where I begin this book when faced with the daunting task of chronicling our lives. How should I portray our journey, through satire or seriousness? In truth, I do not have a definitive answer. Therefore, I will simply start at the beginning, which entails delving into the kind of individual that I am, starting with a brief account of my childhood, and early adult life.

Chapter I

In the Quiet Corner of My Average Existence.

"If I achieve little in life besides being a good father, then I'd have achieved something momentous"- Matthew Ellis

Though my life may not be marked by extraordinary accomplishments or grand ambitions, I have come to realize that being a good father or parent is a profoundly special achievement in itself.

Growing up in the 1980s on a typical working-class suburban council estate of the UK, my childhood was mostly unremarkable. I was reminded from time to time that I was born because of what my parents referred to as a "good mistake." They had married hastily due to my impending arrival, seeking to avoid any stigma associated with being born out of wedlock. Such were the norms of the late 1970s.

During my early years, nothing particularly extraordinary happened. However, there was one thing that stood out: my parents were still figuring out how to be adults themselves. My mom was a teenager, and my dad had just turned 21. It was only natural for them to make some mistakes along the way, but luckily, our extended family members were always there to lend a hand and offer support. This support system played a significant role in shaping my family values and the strong bonds I still cherish today.

When I was around three or four years old, we moved from a small two-bedroom flat to my grandparents' house. It was a much bigger and more spacious place, with two living rooms, multiple bedrooms, and an amazing garden. The house backed onto a beautiful woodland and country park, which became my personal playground. I would spend hours exploring, using my imagination to create all sorts of exciting adventures.

Life was simpler back then in the 1980s, with homemade meals and a limited selection of television channels. Personal computers, video games, and the wonders of the internet were mostly but distant dreams. Entertainment came in the form of children's shows, books, and imaginative play in the great outdoors.

As a young boy, I was captivated by blockbuster movies like Star Wars, Ghostbusters, and The Goonies. These films sparked my imagination and led to endless adventures with my Star Wars action figures, particularly the endearing Ewoks figures. In the garden, I would recreate scenes from the movies, fashioning hideouts for my toy companions among the bushes, with my imagination fuelling problem-solving skills and creativity.

It was during this time that I learned the power of empathy through watching E.T. The Extra-Terrestrial. It was my first cinema experience with my parents, and I still remember having a range of emotions, from relief at the alien's resurrection to sadness at the loss of the bond between the main character and his newfound friend. Empathy and imagination have become invaluable gifts that I have carried with me, yet so young I was unaware of their significance and the impact they would have on my later journeys.

When my younger brother arrived in 1984, I was hoping he'd fulfil my wish for a playmate. However, I soon realized that we had different interests and aspirations, not to mention a five year age gap, which is enormous when you're a child. Little did I know that my brother would also be labelled as atypical, with his own unique traits and challenges that would shape his own path as we grew up together.

As I prepared for secondary school, my mother presented me with an unconventional opportunity. She proposed that I attend a boarding school located outside our local area, believing it would provide better educational opportunities and foster independence at a young age. Intrigued by the prospect, I embraced the change, unaware of the impact it would later have on my relationship with my father.

Being away from home for long periods of time made me realize how much I missed having my father around. His work schedule kept us apart for months on end, and it frustrated me that we couldn't spend more time together. So, I came up with a plan to run away from school and surprise my parents by walking all the way home. But things didn't go as planned. I got lost and ended up in a different town, with no way to contact my parents because mobile phones didn't exist back then. I had to search for a payphone, which was one of the older red box telephones, which you mostly only see in old movies now. I had to make a reverse charge call to let them know where I was, which was difficult to explain as I only had a road name, because like mobile phones there was no GPS or Sat-Navs to guide them to me, but they eventually found me and took me back to school to discuss why I'd left. This incident made me realize just how important my father's role was and how much I missed him during his long absences. It had a lasting impact on me, even as I grew older and eventually became a father myself. The echoes of his absence would resurface in my own journey of fatherhood.

As a young adult, I must admit that I felt a rush to find a partner, get married, establish a home, and conform to society's expectations of a typical family. My parents, who married at a young age due to my impending arrival, serve as an example of this same pattern. While they have successfully maintained their marriage over the course of forty-five years, it hasn't been without its challenges. They possess distinct interests, hobbies, and levels of intellect. As they will likely read this book, it is important to acknowledge their enduring commitment and the family they have built, which includes my brother, myself, and their three grandchildren comprised of my daughter Rose, son Rory, and my nephew.

At twenty-one years old, I entered into marriage feeling a profound sense of accomplishment, deviating from the conventional family tradition of getting married with a child on the way. My wife and I then took the leap and purchased our own house. Four years into our marriage, we received the joyous news of expecting our first child. However, just before our daughter's arrival in August 2004, my beloved great-grandmother passed away. She held the role of a remarkable matriarch within the extended family, connecting its members with love and care. I had a deep bond with her, as she played a significant part in raising me during her retirement years. In her memory, I cherish her teachings, values, and the affection she showered upon me. Her sudden demise from a massive heart attack at the age of eighty-four in May 2004 marked the end of an era. I am grateful that she spent her final afternoon surrounded by family, enjoying a meal of Fish and Chips with my uncle and aunt, and she was grateful for recovering from a recent cold to be able to take the trip out with them.

Three months later, our daughter Rose entered the world, and in honour of my great-grandmother's extraordinary legacy, we bestowed upon her the same name "Rose." Rose, now a young woman herself, embodies the same determination, strong will, and love that characterized her namesake. Though like many young individuals of her generation, she occasionally displays traits of being opinionated, self-absorbed, and entitled. However, her presence in our lives brings immeasurable joy and fulfilment. Little did I know that shortly after Rose's birth, I would face my first encounter with depression. Looking back, I realize it was likely triggered by the combination of losing such an influential family member and the sudden responsibility of nurturing a vulnerable little person in Rose. The arrival of a child swiftly bestowed upon me the

16

virtues of responsibility, patience, and boundless love. Truly, one cannot fully grasp the transformative power of parenthood until experiencing it first-hand. Anyway, that initial episode of depression was thankfully fleeting, unrecognized for what it truly was until many years later.

Five years after Rose's birth, we were blessed with the arrival of our second child, Rory. When he was born, he appeared perfect, although I couldn't help but notice his unusually large hands, which led me to speculate about his future potential as a basketball player or goalkeeper. During Rory's early years, two things stand out in my memory: the sleepless nights he brought upon himself and us, and the fact that his excrement consistently resembled black, pungent pond sludge. Other than the last peculiarity, Rory's first year was, to the best of my recollection, fairly typical.

As I now reflect on the nineteen years of caring for my two children, and particularly Rory over the last thirteen of those, one word encompasses my journey, and that's acceptance. However, for individuals living with those with autism, acquiring this fundamental skill of acceptance can be incredibly challenging for some men or fathers. Having experienced firsthand the lack of fathers attending workshops and seminars on the condition, many mothers have told me that their partner or their child's father seemed to find it difficult to accept or even acknowledge the diagnosis of ASD and the new responsibility and expectations of their child's differences.

I fully accept that Rory and I will always encounter challenges due to his condition, such as his limited diet, preference for wearing blue, or the need to undress into specific clothing at home. In all honesty, if there were a magical pill available today that could eliminate Rory's autism, I wouldn't administer it myself. He should have the autonomy to decide if and when he wants to explore such options when he reaches the appropriate age and capacity. This may sound like an unconventional statement, but the challenges he faces and has already overcome are a result of his unique identity as an autistic individual. It has shaped his character and how he perceives and interacts with the world in his own extraordinary way. Autism should not be equated with conditions like dementia or Alzheimer's, where a person's character maybe changed, forgotten or lost. Instead, autism represents just another way of thinking, perceiving, and overcoming the challenges posed by a neurotypical way of thinking or acting in society.

While attributing modern-day medical conditions to historical figures is speculative, some researchers and historians have suggested that certain individuals from history may have exhibited traits consistent with autism. Examples include:

Albert Einstein:

The renowned physicist's exceptional intelligence and distinctive thought processes have led some to propose that he displayed traits associated with autism, such as social difficulties and repetitive behaviours.

Isaac Newton:

The groundbreaking scientist's intense focus on his work, solitary tendencies, and struggles with social interactions have raised the possibility of him being autistic.

Emily Dickinson:

The American poet's reclusive nature, fascination with particular subjects and routines, and introverted tendencies are characteristics often associated with autism.

Mozart:

The musical prodigy's social awkwardness and repetitive behaviours have sparked speculation about a potential connection to autism.

Andy Warhol:

The famous pop artist's fixation on repetitive patterns and unique communication style have prompted experts to consider the likelihood of being on the spectrum.

Sir Isaac Asimov:

The prolific science fiction writer and biochemist is thought to have exhibited traits consistent with autism, including social challenges and a strong focus on specific subjects.

If any of the aforementioned figures were indeed autistic, wouldn't it have been a great loss to the world and our cultural history if their unique ways of thinking and contributions to society were altered by a magical pill in an attempt to make them more "normal" or neurotypical. Autism has likely existed throughout our past, the present, and in future generations of individuals, and it should not be treated as a problem to be fixed. Instead, it should be accepted, understood, and embraced. Being different doesn't mean being less valuable; it simply means being unique and adding diverse perspectives to our world.

Chapter II

A Brief History of Autism

"If you've met one person with autism, you've met one person with autism."
– Dr Stephen Shore

Early accounts of autism can be traced back to the late 19th century when numerous case studies highlighting children with atypical behaviours and social impairments were documented. One of the earliest descriptions of autism was provided by French psychiatrist Victor Lotte in 1867. Lotte described a boy who exhibited severe social withdrawal, self-injury, and a complete disconnection from the surrounding world. Lotte referred to this condition as "dementia infantilis" or "childhood dementia," recognizing it as a rare and severe form of mental illness.

Other European psychiatrists in the late 19th and early 20th centuries also made early depictions of autism. In 1906, Swiss psychiatrist Eugen Bleuler first employed the term "autism" from the Greek word "autós" meaning 'self' and used to describe the tendency of individuals with schizophrenia to retreat into their own world and lose touch with reality. However, it was not until the 1940s that the term "autism" was specifically used to describe the distinct condition we now identify as autism.

Austrian-American psychiatrist Leo Kanner played a pivotal role in defining autism. In 1943, he published a groundbreaking paper titled "Autistic Disturbances of Affective Contact." Kanner described eleven children who exhibited a unique pattern of behaviour and social impairment, providing the first comprehensive account of autism. He observed a lack of interest in social interaction, repetitive behaviours, limited interests, delayed language development, and difficulty forming emotional connections with others. Kenner's theory of "refrigerator mothers" is a now-discredited hypothesis to explain the causes of autism. The theory suggested that cold and unemotional parenting, particularly from mothers, was responsible for the development of the condition. It implied that a lack of maternal warmth and emotional connection led to the social and behavioural impairments observed in individuals with autism. However, extensive research and understanding of autism have debunked this theory, recognizing that it is instead a complex neurodevelopmental condition with genetic, environmental, and biological origins. Though the notion of "refrigerator mothers" is now discredited, his research recognised the inherent neurological differences and diverse range of factors that contribute to the development of the condition. His paper had at least garnered significant interest among psychiatrists, leading to continued research and treatment of children with the condition. Kanner later refined his understanding of autism in subsequent papers, identifying a broader range of symptoms and characteristics associated with the condition.

Concurrently, another psychiatrist named Hans Asperger in Vienna was studying children with social impairments, particularly what was then termed high-functioning autism. However, Asperger's work initially received limited recognition within the psychiatric community. There have been some historical accounts suggesting that Hans Asperger, may have had some involvement with the Nazi regime during World War II. It is believed that Asperger's work was influenced by the prevailing eugenics ideology of the time, which sought to promote the "purity" of the Aryan race and eliminate individuals deemed undesirable.

While some evidence suggests that Asperger may have cooperated with the Nazi authorities, particularly in relation to the forced sterilization of individuals with disabilities, the extent of his involvement and his personal beliefs remain a subject of debate and ongoing investigation among historians.

So, it is important to note that Asperger's syndrome as a condition is not associated with Nazism or any form of extremism. The syndrome was named after Hans Asperger due to his early research and descriptions of the condition. It is a neurodevelopmental disorder characterized by challenges in social interaction, communication, and restrictive and repetitive patterns of behaviour, and it affects individuals regardless of their race, ethnicity, or political beliefs. It is crucial to separate the individual's historical context from the understanding and recognition of Asperger's syndrome as a valid neurodevelopmental condition. As our understanding of history evolves, it is essential to acknowledge and learn from past mistakes while ensuring that individuals with Asperger's and other autism spectrum disorders are not stigmatized or associated with ideologies or actions, they have no control over.

It was not until the 1980s that Asperger's research gained broader acceptance. In 1981, British psychiatrist Lorna Wing published a paper describing a milder form of autism, which she referred to as "Asperger syndrome." Wing's work popularized the concept of autism as a spectrum, with individuals exhibiting varying degrees of symptom severity.

Another significant milestone in the history of autism was its inclusion in the Diagnostic and Statistical Manual of Mental Disorders (DSM), published by the American Psychiatric Association. The DSM is a widely used classification system for mental disorders, and the inclusion of autism helped establish it as a recognized disorder internationally. The first edition of the DSM, published in 1952, did not include autism as a distinct disorder. However, the second edition, released in 1968, classified autism as a subtype of schizophrenia. This categorization was controversial, as it presumed autism to be a form of childhood psychosis rather than a distinct condition. In 1980, the third edition (DSM-III) introduced autism as a separate disorder for the first time. The diagnostic criteria were based on Kanner's original description and encompassed social impairments, communication difficulties, and repetitive behaviours. This inclusion raised awareness of autism and facilitated formal diagnoses.

Subsequent revisions of the DSM have continued to refine and update the criteria for diagnosing autism. The fourth edition (DSM-IV) introduced the concept of Asperger syndrome as a distinct disorder in 1994. It characterized individuals with social impairments and repetitive behaviours but without significant language or cognitive delays. The fifth & revised edition (DSM-5TR), published in 2022, introduced the category of "autism spectrum disorder" (ASD), consolidating classic (Kanner's) autism, Asperger syndrome, and related conditions.

Medical and social understanding of autism has advanced, theories regarding its underlying causes have also evolved. Early theories focused on psychological and environmental factors, while contemporary research has emphasized biological and neurological factors. The "intense world" theory suggests that individuals with autism experience the world with heightened intensity, leading to sensory overload, social impairments, and repetitive behaviours. Other theories focus on brain development and connectivity, highlighting differences in how the brains of individuals with autism develop and connect in regions involved in social cognition and communication. Genetic studies have also revealed the strong genetic component of autism, although the precise genetic mechanisms remain complex and not yet fully understood.

The historical progression of autism research has paved the way for increased awareness, understanding, and support for individuals on the autism spectrum. Ongoing research continues to deepen our knowledge and inform interventions and therapies that enhance the lives of individuals with the condition.

Chapter III

Rory's Past, Present & Future

"Time is relative; its only worth depends upon what we do as it is passing." - Albert Einstein

Past:

My original concept revolved around chronicling Rory's transformative journey over approximately three decades. This first book aims to recount his childhood experiences, while the second book would delve into his teenage and early adult years, and the third and final instalment will hopefully capture his life as a young adult in his twenties or thirties.

In this initial book, I focus on the last twelve years of Rory's life, which may prove to be the most challenging to write. This difficulty arises from my early struggles with his autism diagnosis, the process of accepting it, and my own personal battle with depression and anxiety during some of those early years.

Present:

The year is now 2023 and Rory has overcome so many challenges since starting this book as a distraction to my continued depression and anxiety in 2016. His social cues and etiquettes, as well as personal hygiene and independence, have all improved, he now uses the toilet and has a bath daily and independently most of the time. As a teenage boy of thirteen, he still enjoys Peppa Pig, Ben and Holly's Little Kingdom, Mickey, and particularly Minnie Mouse, as well as the Toy Story movies. He enjoys cooking and helping with household chores, such as washing up, changing bedcovers, and placing them in the washing machine and then out to dry. He has a wickedly slapstick sense of humour and will often laugh uncontrollably at others' misfortune, though it usually happens to be my misfortune he finds the funniest.

For all his advancements though, he's still massively behind his peers of a similar age, and I often refer to him as my "Peter Pan" in the context of his autism and global developmental delay. The comparison to Peter Pan as "the boy who never grew up" may take on some additional layers of meaning. Like Peter Pan, Rory can sometimes display a certain innocence and childlike wonder that persists beyond the typical age of his development. He will often engage in activities or interests that are more characteristic of younger children, demonstrating a timeless quality to his behaviours and interests.

For some autistic children like Rory with developmental delays, their preference for familiar routines and interests might be a way of coping with the challenges they face in the real world. Just as Peter Pan escapes to Neverland to avoid the responsibilities of adulthood, autistic children might retreat into their comfort zones as a coping mechanism for dealing with the complexities and difficulties they encounter in everyday life. For Rory, this is often his bedroom. Both Rory and some other autistic children may fear change and have difficulty adapting to new situations or expectations. The idea of growing up and facing the uncertainties that come with it might be overwhelming for them, leading them to cling to their familiar worlds and the characters that inhabit their lives. Those characters namely being you, I, extended family members, and some social and academic individuals in what could be described as support or dependency networks. Moreover, just as Peter Pan celebrates the power of imagination, many autistic children have rich and vivid imaginations. Their imaginative play might be an essential aspect of

26

their development and communication, providing an avenue for them to express themselves and explore their thoughts and feelings. Additionally, for some autistics, certain environments or activities may serve as a "Neverland" of sorts—a special place where they feel safe, secure, and understood. This place could be a favourite room, a particular activity, or any context where they can fully be themselves without judgment or pressure to conform. While it's essential to recognize that each child's experience is unique and not all autistic children with developmental delays will relate to the Peter Pan analogy. Though my comparison may help highlight some common experiences and characteristics shared by certain autistic individuals, we as caregivers, teachers, and advocates, should understand that these connections can offer insights into how to support and nurture their development in a sensitive and positive manner.

Future:

I only have to remember back three years ago to recall the lack of social interaction and support by the social welfare and care services towards our elderly, infirm and most vulnerable, as those services came under immense strain during the COVID-19 crisis of 2020. What if the next pandemic has a higher rate of transmission or mortality. Worse still what if society broke down entirely due to war or due to extreme and catastrophic long-term weather and climate events. The likely first things to be cut or removed would be social welfare support and similar services. In the US, its estimated that over the next ten years, 707,000 to 1,116,000 teenagers with autism will transition into adulthood and age out of school-based autism support services.

Autistic teens receive healthcare transition services only half as often as those with other special healthcare needs, and those with additional medical issues linked to autism receive even less support during this critical period. Many young adults with autism face a gap

27

in healthcare as they stop seeing paediatricians and do not receive adequate medical attention for years. In the two years following high school, over half of young adults with autism remain unemployed and not enrolled in higher education. This rate is even lower than young adults in other disability categories such as learning disabilities, intellectual disability, or speech-language impairment.

Among the nearly 18,000 individuals with autism who utilized state-funded vocational rehabilitation programs in 2014, only 60 percent were able to secure employment. Of these employed individuals, 80 percent worked part-time, earning a median weekly rate of $160, placing them well below the poverty level. Moreover, nearly half of 25-year-olds with autism have never held a paying job. Though research highlights the significance of job activities that promote independence, as they have been shown to reduce autism symptoms and enhance daily living skills in individuals with autism.

Due to the likely challenges in the future related to social welfare funding and availability uncertainties within the UK welfare system, we have made the decision to relocate. We will be joining other family members, specifically my parents, on a smallholding in Scotland. This move is intended to provide an alternative to the oversubscribed and underfunded services in our densely populated Essex town, situated on the borders of Greater London. Our plan is to wait until Rory reaches the age of nineteen and completes his special needs education (SEN).

During this time, we aim to teach him how to sustainably and self-sufficiently manage the smallholding, which will involve keeping livestock and cultivating his own produce. As a preliminary step, we have already introduced twenty-two chickens, several beehives, and cultivated fruit and vegetable patches in our mid-terraced suburban home in our bustling Essex town. The overarching goal is to scale up these efforts in the future to help mitigate the rising social costs associated with food and energy prices, all while providing Rory with a sense of purpose through productive work and allowing him to witness the tangible results of his and our efforts. Thus, we plan to educate him to live semi-independently within an annex, self-contained cabin, or static home on the same property where Jennifer, I, and his grandparents reside. Rory will also assist me with the smallholding tasks until he becomes proficient enough to manage them independently, with the potential to achieve full independence when Jennifer and I are no longer there to guide him.

Nevertheless, this decision to prioritize Rory's safety by relocating in the future could potentially limit his ability to form social connections if we choose a secluded and isolated location. It might deprive him of friendships and even romantic relationships. However, at this point, the future remains uncertain, and I hope to document our next chapter in a follow-up book in the next five to six years after we have relocated. Until then, I will strive not to overly worry about the future, as dwelling on it can be both stressful and emotionally taxing. My imagination sometimes fills in the gaps of Rory's life when Jennifer and I are no longer around to care for his well-being. This, I know, is the most significant fear shared by almost every parent or caregiver of an autistic or disabled loved one—the fear of the unknown once we are gone.

Unfortunately, the likely outcomes for severely autistic adults in the future, based on the UK social system, can vary significantly, as each person's situation is unique. However, several common factors influence their prospects.

Limited Independence:

Many severely autistic adults will continue to require significant support and assistance to meet their daily living needs. The level of independence achieved may vary, but most will likely rely on some form of caregiving or assistance throughout their lives.

Social Isolation:

The lack of understanding and awareness about autism in society may lead to social isolation for these individuals. Social opportunities and connections might be limited, which can impact their overall well-being and mental health.

Employment Challenges:

Finding and maintaining meaningful employment can be extremely challenging for severely autistic adults. The job market may struggle to accommodate their specific needs and capabilities, leading to high levels of unemployment or underemployment.

Housing and Accommodation:

The availability of suitable housing and accommodation options tailored to the needs of severely autistic adults may be limited. This could result in long waiting lists for appropriate facilities, or individuals may end up in environments that are not fully equipped to meet their requirements.

Family Support:

Families often play a critical role in supporting severely autistic adults. However, as parents and caregivers age, the burden of care may shift to other family members or the social care system, potentially leading to additional challenges in providing adequate support.

Access to Services:

The availability and quality of social and healthcare services for severely autistic adults can vary across regions in the UK. Accessibility to specialized therapies, education, and support may be limited, leading to disparities in outcomes.

Financial Concerns:

The cost of providing lifelong care and support for severely autistic adults can be financially burdensome for families and the social system. Budget constraints may affect the level of care and support provided.

Vulnerability:

Severely autistic adults may be more vulnerable to exploitation and abuse due to their communication difficulties and dependence on others for care. Safeguarding measures must be in place to protect their well-being.

While the UK social system strives to provide support and services for autistic individuals, including severe cases, there are ongoing challenges to address. Improving awareness, increasing funding for specialized services, and promoting inclusive policies can enhance the outlook for severely autistic adults and their families in the future.

Chapter IV

Diagnosis

"I am different, not less" – Dr Temple Gradin

In the early years, it was not immediately apparent that my Rory was different, or as I prefer to say nowadays, unique. As a baby, he exhibited the expected giggles and laughter at everyday sounds and actions. However, one noticeable difference was the pungent odour and consistency of his stools, which resembled pond water. I wondered if he might be lactose intolerant or have some undiagnosed dietary requirement. Our doctor reassured us that despite the loose stools, Rory was still gaining weight and appeared healthy. Though as Rory approached his first birthday, he had not yet learned to walk or even attempt to stand.

Considering that we already had a neurotypical daughter Rose, I subscribed to the belief that girls develop faster than boys, we attributed Rory's delay to his gender. Instead of crawling, Rory shuffled along on his bum, which amused us and made me think he was an adaptable boy finding an alternative method that worked for him. And indeed, it did. However, by around eighteen months, his vocabulary and mobility had not progressed, causing both ourselves and his nursery to become concerned that something may be amiss. We were referred to a paediatrician at our local clinic.

The clinician, like others before, assured us that there was likely no cause for worry and that boys may simply take longer to reach certain milestones. Drawing from her own experience as a mother, she shared that her son had also bum shuffled and that it was merely a sign of laziness. While Rory had started attempting to pull himself up and we had introduced a walker and bouncer at home, he seemed increasingly unhappy and clingy. I attributed this to his frustration at being unable to keep pace with his peers at nursery or even his sister at home. During this time, he sought extra reassurance and sought the constant company of his mother. He became what some refer to as a "mummy's boy" between the ages of two and three.

Additionally, he refused to sleep in his own cot bed, often waking up at all hours of the night and morning. Life during those years was incredibly challenging for everyone as he would become upset seemingly without reason. Little did I know at the time, as I will later explain in the chapter on behaviour. Is that all behaviour is a form of communication, much like a baby crying. A baby cries because it has no other means to communicate its needs, whether it's hunger, discomfort, pain, or simply the desire for affection and reassurance. Crying is its most effective means of expression. Though it is also true that if a baby cries for an extended period without receiving attention, it may learn to stop crying altogether.

Around this time, I also noticed that Rory seemed disinterested in his toys and puzzles, except for one particular toy he received for Christmas in 2011. It was a toy where you placed a Ping-Pong ball in a pipe at the top, and a cushion of air pushed the ball through the tubing, popping out in an adjacent hole before repeating the process. Rory found immense joy in this repetitive play, accompanied by smiles and giggles that were wonderful to witness. It was during this time that he started flapping his hands in a comical manner. Unbeknownst to us, this flapping was a form of stimulation, or "stim/stimming" often associated with individuals on the spectrum. The repetitive nature of the ball traversing the tubes and the cause-and-effect sequence delighted him. Later, I noticed this repetitive behaviour in other areas of Rory's life, such as when he wanted to be picked up and to switch the lights on and off repeatedly until I stopped the activity. I termed this behaviour "cause and effect play," similar to the mentioned ball toy or even when Rory would throw a tennis ball to the dog, engaging in a game that could continue almost indefinitely, providing pleasure to both Rory and our dog Poppy alike.

We later took him for the usual routine and age-related check-up at the local health centre, and it was during that check-up, that the health visitor conducted various tests. One was having Rory pick up small items and, in this instance, and as a reward for cooperating he was handed some 'Smarties' a chocolate treat about the size of a typical shirt button. Yet, Rory as much as he tried to grab them, he was unable to take them when offered, and he couldn't complete the task which was tried several times. The clinician then seemed a little concerned, as Rory was showing less dexterity than he should for his age. We were asked to bring him back for a second review, which led to a referral to a consultant paediatrician. Soon after, we met a kind and relaxed paediatric consultant who preferred not to make hasty judgments. After his initial assessment, he decided to monitor Rory's progress and also mentioned Dyspraxia and global developmental delay (GDD), though at the time I had little idea what these were, but the paediatrician stated Rory's future development would soon indicate a likely outcome. I came away feeling confused and shocked.

It was now summertime, and Rory was now almost two years of age. We decided to go on a family camping holiday, all I remember from that trip was Rory being extremely stressed, often throwing tantrums, and screaming on the floor, needing constant attention and endless books or one of our mobile phones just to keep him engaged for a few minutes before seemingly becoming upset again, with nothing able to pacify him for the duration of that holiday. Over the course of the next few months, Rory underwent a complete transformation. He had excessive tantrums and regressed in social interactions. What limited development was made with his speech was slowing down or had stopped, and it became difficult to participate in the songs he used to enjoy. Rory seemed to drift away, leaving us with a stressed, and disconnected child a lot of the time.

It wouldn't be until the age of three and a half before Rory received an official diagnosis, but during that time, we had regular visits with clinicians, social care, and hospitals and the diagnosis eventually felt like a formality, yet a huge relief to so many mounting questions during Rory's development or lack there of.

As parents our worries and focus were on Rory, wondering how his condition would impact his life or our lives. In our research of the condition, we came across information about autism at various points on the spectrum, but at the time, it all felt to alien, and I remember feeling a sense of detachment from discussing or acknowledging my son could be or was different in anyway.

Looking back, I can now recognise early signs of developmental delay in Rory, although I didn't realise it at the time. As a young parent, I relied on my parents and in particular my own mother's knowledge and experience to track their milestones, but even those didn't raise any concerns for me. It's only with hindsight that I can now connect the dots and see the numerous indicators that were present. When asking about autism in our family's history, the official answer is no. However, I now recognize many autistic traits in my ex-wife's uncle, my own uncle, and even myself being neurodivergent although there is no established diagnosis to support it. Rory is the first to be formally diagnosed in our family, and it's not uncommon for parents and relatives of diagnosed children to subsequently receive an autism spectrum diagnosis themselves. Many adults have developed their own coping strategies without fully understanding their difficulties until a younger family member is diagnosed, shedding new light on the family dynamics. Family history may provide some indication, but it's not a reliable test as diagnoses continue to evolve. There are many curiosities from my childhood that bring into question my own neurotype, but at middle age and with a moderately happy and successful life any form of diagnosis would have little impact for me now.

Before having Rory, I had no knowledge of autism beyond the movie 'Rainman' starring Dustin Hoffman as the titular character, with Tom Cruise as his neuro-typical brother. My only real introduction to autism came through Rory and from the internet, as I didn't have family members to turn to for answers. Both sides of the family have since been on a learning curve and the same journey of discovery together.

When an acquaintance recently asked the cause of Rory's autism, it was such a complex question with no definitive answer for me to give. I believe that autism maybe the result of a genetic predisposition inherited from both my ex-wife and/or myself. However, there are almost certainly other variables at play that influence the extent of his symptoms, as yet some hypotheses are speculative, though raise important questions about the role of environment and external factors in autism development. For instance, in the late 1990's to early 2000's the topic of vaccinations was a sensitive one for parents of children with autism. I've read some research papers on the falsely claimed link between the MMR vaccine and autism and feel saddened by how one scientist's erroneous claims garnered more attention than the countless validated studies.

We are seeing the same again in modern day having just come out of Covid-19 and the inevitable good that the covid vaccine did. Despite this, the question of whether to vaccinate children remains in every parent's mind. Both of my children were vaccinated, and I firmly believe that vaccines themselves do not cause or are connected to autism. However, there are concerns about whether multiple vaccinations could potentially harm children with known developmental health conditions. Vaccines are typically administered on developing individuals and not vulnerable members of society. I believe it's crucial to examine how vaccinations are offered and whether they might affect individuals with pre-existing medical conditions. In Rory's case, we decided that the benefits of the MMR vaccine outweighed the associated risks and complications of measles, mumps or rubella might have on him in later life.

In the UK, the resurgence of measles and the low uptake of crucial vaccinations have reinforced my confidence in the decision to vaccinate my children. I would be devastated to realize that my choice not to vaccinate could have detrimental effects on other families. This raises the question of whether vaccination is solely a personal decision or a wider social responsibility.

I also understand that this topic may evoke various emotions and opinions, and it's a complex issue that requires careful consideration.

Post Diagnosis Support

For me after having my world turned upside down, I was in a daze. I had little idea where to start besides being handed a leaflet about autism from the consultant paediatrician, but here in the United Kingdom, there are a variety of support services for families with autistic children, encompassing educational support, financial assistance, health and social care, and community resources. These services aim to help families navigate the challenges associated with raising a child with ASD, but ultimately won't prepare you for the experience, but here is a brief overview of the support available:

Educational Support:

- Special Educational Needs and Disability (SEND) Support: Local authorities are responsible for identifying and providing support to children with special educational needs and disabilities, including autism. This can involve additional classroom assistance, specialized equipment, and adaptations to the curriculum.

- Education, Health, and Care (EHC) Plans: For children with complex needs, an EHC plan can be created to outline the support they require across education, health, and social care.

Financial Support:

- Disability Living Allowance (DLA): Designed for individuals with disabilities, including autism, DLA assists with the extra costs associated with care and mobility. It consists of a care component and a mobility component.

- Personal Independence Payment (PIP): Similar to DLA, PIP aids adults aged 16-64 with long-term health conditions or disabilities, including autism. It is divided into a daily living component and a mobility component.

- Carer's Allowance: Available to those caring for individuals with disabilities or health conditions, including children with autism, this benefit requires a minimum of 35 hours of care per week.

Health and Social Care:

- Health Services: The National Health Service (NHS) provides various services for children with autism, including specialized assessments, speech and language therapy, occupational therapy, and mental health support.

- Social Care: Local authorities assess and offer support to families with disabled children, which can include assistance with daily living, respite care, and home adaptations.

Community Resources:

- Support Groups: Families can access online or in-person support groups where they can connect with other parents, share experiences and advice, and gather information and resources.

- Advocacy Services: Available advocacy services help families navigate the support system and access necessary services, providing guidance on education, social care, and benefits.

- Leisure Activities: Programs such as sports and arts groups offer leisure activities tailored for children with autism, fostering social skills development, self-confidence, and enjoyment.

- Respite Care: Families can benefit from respite care, which provides temporary relief from caregiving responsibilities through day services or overnight stays in residential settings.

The specific support available depends on the individual needs of the child and family. It is crucial for families to seek information and support from various sources, such as local authorities, health and social care services, and advocacy and support groups. But one significant challenge faced by families and individuals with autism is the lack of adequate funding for autistic resources. Despite the increased recognition and understanding of autism as a prevalent neurodevelopmental condition, the allocation of funds for essential support services and resources often falls short of meeting the growing demand.

One area where the impact of limited funding is felt is in the education system. Many schools struggle to provide the specialized support and accommodations necessary for children to thrive academically and socially. Insufficient funding often translates into larger class sizes, a lack of specialized staff, and limited access to tailored educational programs. As a result, children with autism may not receive the individualized attention and interventions they require, which can impede their educational progress and overall well-being.

Another area greatly affected by the funding gap is healthcare. While the National Health Service (NHS) provides vital services for individuals with autism, such as diagnostic assessments and some therapies, there is often a significant wait time for these services due to limited resources. Moreover, access to specialized interventions, such as speech and language therapy, may be limited or inaccessible due to long waiting lists or high costs. The lack of funding and resources puts additional strain on families who are already navigating the complex challenges, making it difficult to access the comprehensive care and support their loved ones need.

The shortage of funding also impacts community resources and support networks for individuals and their families. Community-based organizations and charities that provide invaluable services, such as support groups, respite care, and recreational activities, often struggle to secure sufficient funding to meet the growing demand. As a result, families may face limited options for connecting with others who share similar experiences, accessing respite services, or participating in inclusive community programs.

The consequences of insufficient funding for autistic resources are far-reaching and affect autistic individuals, as well as their families across various aspects of their lives.

Chapter V

The Measure of a Man

"It is not possible to produce a set of rules to describe what a man should do in every conceivable set of circumstances"- Alan Turing

We humans are distinct from other great apes in several significant ways. While we share a common ancestry and are closely related, there are notable differences that set us apart in our form of social structures and that of communication.

Social Structures:

Human societies are characterized by complex social structures and institutions, involving intricate networks of relationships and cooperation. We engage in various forms of social organization, including kinship systems, economic systems, governance structures, and religious institutions. Our societies exhibit a higher degree of specialization, division of labour, and cultural diversity compared to other great ape societies.

Communication and Language:

While other great apes possess communication systems and can convey basic information, human language is far more sophisticated and complex. Humans can express an extensive range of ideas, emotions, and abstract concepts through spoken and written language. Our linguistic abilities facilitate collective learning, collaboration, and the transmission of knowledge.

It is important to note that these differences should not be interpreted as hierarchical or indicative of superiority. Each species, including great apes, has its own unique adaptations and ecological niche.

While humans have distinct attributes, we are part of the larger family of primates and share a common evolutionary heritage with other great apes.

But even in the twenty first century there are still certain expectations to being a man, with a google search of the phrase *"What does it mean to be a man"* returning websites phrases of tough, mean, strong. The Urban Dictionary definition is as follows - *"A man who embodies strength and masculinity, actively pursuing, defending, conquering, and asserting authority."* This definition could almost be the description of the attributes of an alpha male Silverback Gorilla couldn't it.

So for those who don't know the true me have in the past described me as a "mans, man" with my character similar to that of the urban dictionary, but that really isn't the real me because much of what others perceive is merely a façade and the front I portray to the world, because I grew up in a generation where to show emotion, empathy and sentiment was still a sign of weakness.

To understand this better, let's delve back into my childhood. I grew up under the influence of three very strong female figures: my mother, my aunt and my paternal great grandmother. They instilled in me the importance of standing up for myself, advocating for retaliation if attacked. "Never strike first, but always strike back," my mother would say. She justified this by citing the biblical principle of "an eye for an eye, a tooth for a tooth." My grandmother took it a step further, advising me to confront and strike the leader if I encountered a gang. "Punch him where it hurts the most," she would say, mentioning a soapbox, the meaning of which still eludes me to this day, but I think she meant the mouth?

Even though I engaged in activities like Karate, Judo and Rugby, I also enjoyed museum visits and outings with my great grandmother, which was where I learned most of my domestic skills, such as cooking, cleaning, and ironing. In my teenage years, I never dabbled in excessive drinking or drug use, nor did I exhibit overt sexism or misogyny. Instead, I worried about others' perceptions of my character, often empathizing too much instead of living in the moment like my friends. Speaking of friends, most of them remained mere acquaintances after I left boarding school. This pattern still holds true in my life, except for one close friend Bryan that I mentioned at the start of the book. I've always found solace and contentment in my own imagination and solitude.

However, one aspect of my character that has remained consistent from perhaps spending so much time in my youth with strong independent women is that of my empathetic nature. I tend to be emotionally moved and tear up at both major and minor achievements of my children. It's also not uncommon for me to become a blubbering mess while watching emotional movies like "Marley and Me" or "The Green Mile." I simply seem to amplify my emotional connection to what's visually set before me, even though it deviated from societal expectations for boys and men of my era.

Another enduring characteristic of mine is a strong sense of moral responsibility. When I witness someone being unjustly targeted, I often intervene or act as a mediator. My mother proudly recalls an incident when we were walking together and witnessed boys teasing and attempting to steal an old man's walking stick. Though I only vaguely remember the event's details, I apparently shouted at the boys, demanding that they leave the man alone. They promptly fled, and the man expressed his gratitude to both my mother and I. We continued walking together to the shops before parting ways.

However, in life, no matter how diplomatic one may be, there are individuals who relish arguments or engage in bullying. In such cases, I often say, "A bully only understands a bigger bully." This doesn't necessarily imply resorting to physical confrontation, as most bullies today hide behind their phones and keyboards to troll and belittle others, shielded by the safety and anonymity of their home and four walls. Unfortunately, as parents of autistic children, we may experience adverse behaviour or bullying first hand, as some people judge us based on our child's perceived challenging behaviours when out in public spaces. A few may even have the audacity to confront us directly, though most will mutter under their breath or express their opinions on social media. In such situations, it's crucial to limit our social media contacts. In truth, how many true friends do we really have that we need to stay in contact with on social media? It should only be those who have stood by us through thick and thin, aware of our deepest fears and vulnerabilities that are the true friends to hold onto. My advice would be to instead use social media as a tool to connect with others in a similar situation as ourselves, so that when we need to vent after a stressful day, it's often best to seek solace among fellow parents and caregivers who may share our experiences, as they have likely traversed a similar path or are still walking it alongside us, and hopefully offering understanding of the hardships we face.

Interestingly, I've found that women are particularly adept at comprehending and empathizing when I discuss my parenting struggles. On numerous occasions, women have remarked that I "think like a woman" or "a woman would say that." This sentiment sharply contrasts with the "Man's man" comments I've received from male associates. This topic leads me to reflect on my perception of the modern man's role in parenting, and how attitudes and outlooks have evolved over the past decade from traditional father's roles, of often limited to being the breadwinner and providing financial support for the family, while the mother took on the primary responsibility for child-rearing. Certainly, the end of the twentieth century we've seen shifts, changing gender roles, and evolving family dynamics have now led to a transformation in the involvement of fathers and partners in raising children, with some of the key changes being increased participation of fathers and partners now more actively involved in all aspects of child upbringing, including those of caregiving, nurturing, and emotional support. As us fathers take on a greater share of parenting responsibilities, such as feeding, bathing, playing, and attending to the child's needs, fostering a more egalitarian approach to parenting.

Below, I highlight some of the shifts we have witnessed in the UK during my lifetime and in 2023, which are in stark contrast to those of my own father's role some forty plus years ago:

Shared Parental Leave:

Many Western European countries have implemented policies promoting shared parental leave, allowing both parents to take time off work to care for their newborn or young child. This shift acknowledges the importance of fathers and partners in early child development and supports their active involvement from the earliest stages of a child's life.

Changing Gender Roles:

Western European societies have witnessed a gradual erosion of traditional gender roles which was particularly true both during and proceeding the second world war, with my great grandmother being one of those women working within a male dominated work role on the railways. The transition was gradual, but more women are pursuing careers now and more men embracing caregiving roles than a century ago. This shift has allowed fathers, to actively participate in child upbringing and share household responsibilities, challenging traditional gender norms.

Increased Emphasis on Emotional Bonding:

I know this to be true and it wasn't more obvious to me than after my ex-wife and I first separated. My ex-wife and children would remain within the family home to retain stability for both children's development, and in particularly the need to keep Rory's environment and routines as unchanged as possible. So, I would

45

have the children every rest day and holiday that I could at Jennifers flat, but whenever it was time for Rory to return home to his mother his behaviour became more erratic and unpredictable.

Fathers and partners are now encouraged to develop strong emotional bonds with their children. This involves active engagement in activities that promote emotional connection, such as reading to the child, playing, and engaging in open and supportive communication. The recognition of the importance of father-child bonding has led to a more holistic approach to parenting.

Recognition of Paternal Involvement:

Take it from me as the now full-time carer to both my children, that the impact I have had on them, and them me, and that of my own mental wellbeing cannot be over emphasized. There is growing recognition of the positive impact of fathers and partners on child development and well-being. Research has shown that children benefit from the active involvement of fathers and partners in terms of cognitive development, emotional stability, and social skills. This recognition has contributed to the societal shift in attitudes towards the role of fathers and partners in child upbringing.

The shift in the child's upbringing in Western Europe has now evolved from a traditional breadwinner role to one of active involvement, emotional support, and shared responsibility, and reflects a more egalitarian approach to parenting and an understanding of the importance of both parents' contributions in raising healthy and well-adjusted children. But, while gender equality between the sexes has made progress, there is still work to be done. If you were to ask a group of teenagers, both male and female, about their future roles as family members, most would likely echo the traditional narrative that has been ingrained in us through societal norms, media, and even education. This narrative often still portrays the mother as the primary caregiver and nurturer, while the father is seen as the provider, and often less attuned to the child's emotional needs due to spending less time in the family home.

In our modern society, it is imperative that men and fathers no longer adhere to outdated notions of male chauvinism. The roles of men and fathers should no longer mimic the dominance of the alpha silverback gorilla, but instead embrace equality with mothers. Men should play an equal part in providing financial stability while also taking on the role of caregiver and the associated responsibilities and bonding that come with it. This transformation is essential because women have evolved far beyond just being mothers. They earned the right to vote in 1928 and ventured into traditionally male-dominated fields, particularly during the World War I and II efforts. Women have fought for and achieved strides towards equal pay and benefits in many professions, a change that is both just and long overdue.

So, rather than putting up a facade of being a stereotypical 'man's man,' it is crucial to lead by example in the care and upbringing of our children. By doing so, you not only contribute to their well-being but also set a positive precedent for future generations. Remember, the world is changing, and one day, your child may be the one taking care of you. Embracing equality and sharing parenting responsibilities will not only strengthen your family but also contribute to a more progressive and equitable society where everyone's contributions are valued and respected.

Chapter VI

There's Nothing Wrong!

"If you're that depressed, reach out to someone. And remember, suicide is a permanent solution, to a temporary problem."- Robin Williams

As mentioned in a previous chapter when Rory was around two years old and attending nursery, we'd noticed something might be different, so he was undergoing medical investigation at that time, and since I was still working as a postman and had more flexibility in my schedule, I was then the primary caregiver for our children. This allowed me to finish work early in the afternoon and pick up Rory from nursery, followed by his older sister from school.

Over that past year or so, Rory's behaviour at the nursery had become a cause for concern. It became a regular occurrence for me to receive calls at work asking me to pick up Rory early due to issues like not settling, hurting himself, or hurting other children. He would pull other children's hair or bite them, and when he got upset with himself, he would throw himself backward and hit his head on the floor repeatedly. Sometimes, we could identify triggers for these behaviours, but most of the time, I would make excuses like "he must be tired" or "he gets easily frustrated." However, as the months went by and the incidents became more frequent and intense, the nursery management suggested that it might be helpful to involve social services or other agencies that dealt with childhood development, as Rory was not meeting the expected milestones in areas like talking, reading, or writing. I would dismiss this by attributing it to him being a boy and slower than his sister, who had previously attended the same nursery before starting school.

Honestly, I didn't want to admit that Rory might be different in any way, and I definitely didn't want someone who didn't know him as well as we did to label him in any manner. In my eyes, Rory was just an energetic, rough-and-tumble boy who was a little behind his peers. After all, he had started walking late, not finding his balance and coordination until he was almost two years old. He was simply a late bloomer who would catch up in his own time.

It was later arranged for a family key worker to visit the nursery, observe Rory, and discuss any concerns with the staff and management. If any significant issues were found, we would be informed, along with the nursery, and further recommendations and referrals were likely to follow.

For almost ten years as a postman, everything had been relatively well. I enjoyed my job and cherished the moments I could share with my children. But as time went on, things began to change. My working hours became less accommodating, and I started having conflicts with my bosses. Eventually, it all came crashing down, and I was fired from my job. It was a sudden decision I made to hold onto the mail for a couple days, an acted termed 'Wilful delay' by Royal Mail and is a sackable offence. I was hoping to provide stability for my youngest son Rory who was going through a tough time at nursery that week. Little did I know that, that action would lead to grave consequences and my imminent dismissal, shattering the routine I had worked so hard to establish for my family.

It was during this period; I also began to notice problems in my marriage. After nearly ten years of being together and having two amazing, but distinct, children, the strain of losing my job and the ongoing challenges we had with Rory started to affect my mental well-being and relationship. Looking back now, I realize that I tied the knot way too early, at the age of 21. Like my parents' own experience of getting married quickly, I still had a lot of self-discovery and life lessons to learn. However, I don't regret those years at all. They played a significant role in shaping the person I am today and took me on a life journey that I could never have envisioned when I was younger.

As the months went by, the nursery's concerns and complaints grew stronger, and my wife was becoming upset with the constant remarks about seeking help or a referral. She would often get emotional and ask, "Why is it always Rory?" or, like me, say, "He's just lazier than his sister was." But as time passed and we saw the gap in social development between Rory and his peers, we began to question our own beliefs. Rory was also becoming more physically challenging for his mother as he started walking and would resist going to certain places like shopping malls, supermarkets, and even the nursery. Of course, he couldn't communicate verbally yet, so his only way of expressing himself was through physical outbursts. So, reluctantly, when Rory was around two years old, we decided to accept the nursery's recommendation and seek help from child services.

That very first report of that visit is here in its entirety, but for the sake of privacy of individuals, names have been changed-

- *On arrival Rory was singing with a member of staff, filling in the missing words. Kelsey said he is engaging more in activities spending periods of time at the mega blocks.*

- *Rory has developed a fascination of doors and locks, they redirect Rory's attention to an activity, that using locks in a positive way.*

- *He is demanding attention from a member of staff. He has not been using the 'now and then' board but has been using visual key cards.*

- *He does use them to request what he wants, it should be used to direct what you want him to do, so not him controlling the situation.*

- *If Rory does not want to go somewhere or do something with a different member of staff he will drop to the floor.*

- *Nikki left Rory to play with another child, Rory stood observing and then gradually sat down and began to build with the mega blocks. He is playing alongside Danni, when he throws toys Danni, says stop, he attempts to hit her, Danni stops him, and he does take notice.*

- *Rory builds a tower, Danni begins to develop his concept of turn taking, Danni says "Danni turn" wait and he waits for her to put a brick on. Then Rory turn. Rory does occasionally glance at other children's buildings. He is praised for good waiting when he waits for Debbie to have her turn. Another child (Isabel) is then asked if she wants to play and put a brick on the house.*

- *"Isabel's turn" Rory allowed her to put a brick on the tower. In the middle of playing with the bricks he turns to get the attention of Nikki.*

- *Danni uses the picture of the play dough to get Rory to play with something else. He immediately went to get Nikki, he was spoken to firmly, He did refuse, however it was explained to him what he needs to do and taken to the play dough.*

- *He gestures to go back to Nikki; Danni confirms again first play dough then bricks.*

- *Rory does play with the play dough, using the rolling pin. However, keeps requesting Nikki.*

- *While at the activities, use the time to encourage language and social skills, singing songs, talking about what he is doing, e.g., Rolling, blue bus. Also say one more then finish to give warning of changing an activity.*

- *He then throws a toy in protest of what he is being asked to do. Tell him to pick up the car, if needed, point towards the car to use gesture to what you are saying.*

- *Throughout activities he keeps asking for Nicole and looks over to see where she is? Danni says Nikki working -Rory drawing. He asks to put his picture in his bag, develop his independence by encouraging him to put his own picture away, with support.*

- *When another child went to put a car down a ramp, Rory went to hit his hand out the way, he did however look for an adult for a reaction.*

- *During snack time, he is encouraged to sit on the carpet, he does appear to sit well, listening to the register, it would benefit him having a visual card to show washing hands, register, snack times.*

- *Rory empties the milk cartons after snack time, this could be used as an opportunity to talk to him, socialise with another child.*

Suggestions

- *Use now and then board with pictures to encouraging him to do directed activities, have activities that he may not normally chose to do as well as ones he does, to develop variety and broader knowledge and skills. Including snack, tidy up time.*

- *Always give a warning before changing activities, one more go then finished. Few minutes at activities does not have to be for too long.*

- *During activities use the opportunity to develop his language and social skills, encourage turn taking, (my turn your turn) and interaction with others, learning play skills.*

- *Be firm with what you want him to do if he does not go over to the activity, you want him to do ensure that you reinforce what you want, show him the picture again, take him by the hand towards it.*

- *During circle time, refocus Rory when he gets distracted.*

- *Danni to look for a fidget mat, for times of sitting.*

Looking back now, I realize that receiving that email was just the beginning of numerous series of similar messages and transcripts to come over the years. However, at the time, I was in denial about Rory being different. I thought he was just being uncooperative and independent, struggling to get along with others. I ignored other signs, like his fascination with everyday objects and his lack of speech development.

Over the next year, I gained new employment, and along with Rory's mother we continued to attend various appointments with professionals and specialists. Tests were conducted, assessments were made, and I tried to convince myself that there was still nothing different about Rory. I believed his emotional outbursts during visits to hospitals and health centres were merely acts of seeking attention. Little did I understand then that every behaviour, whether positive or inappropriate, is a form of communication and he was generally communicating his dislike for this change in routine and/or different environment. For Rory, these behaviours signalled distress and discomfort, but we didn't know that at the time.

As Rory approached the age to transition from nursery to school, it became evident that a mainstream school wouldn't provide the necessary support and interaction he needed. We were advised to consider special schools, known as SEN schools, which catered to children with special educational needs. Still in denial, I resisted accepting that my son was different from other boys. We explored different schools and found one that offered a mix of mainstream and additional support. The latter seemed like the ideal choice, as it provided extra assistance while allowing Rory to pursue academic achievements like his sister. However, my expectations for Rory's future and his actual academic abilities and social challenges were far apart, a reality that would later hit me hard when he was eventually permanently excluded from that particular academic setting.

During this period of uncertainty regarding Rory's education and our daughter's transition to secondary school, my wife and I separated. I had been growing distant, emotional, and irrational, feeling lost and wanting to escape from it all. At 30 odd years old, my life was far from the idyllic perfect family unit I had envisioned it would be when I had married. My mental health suffered, but I pretended to be fine, hiding my exhaustion and working more than ever. I regret that for about eighteen months, I would leave my children on a Wednesday night for work and not return home until Sunday evening, too drained and irritable to engage with anyone.

During one of these extended work periods, and overwhelmed by exhaustion, I even contemplated taking my own life. The idea of death seemed like an escape from responsibilities as a parent and from facing the mistakes I had made. I felt constant guilt at this time, guilt for not acknowledging the challenges my son had endured, the challenges he was still likely to endure, and my absence in the family unit. But a moment of clarity, high up on a radio tower mast, made me think of Rory again and his needs. I broke down in tears, realizing the gravity of what I had almost done. This wasn't the last encounter I would have with thoughts of suicide, but at that time, I still didn't understand what was wrong with me.

Depression had gradually taken hold of me, and I lacked the knowledge and awareness to recognize it. I believed it was just a weakness that I needed to overcome. Little did I know, it had started when I lost my job at Royal Mail, which had dramatically changed our family's routines and structure. And I still blamed myself for it all.

Chapter VII

Relationships Part 1

"There are times when two people need to step apart from one another, but there is no rule that says they have to turn and fire." - Robert Brault

Marital/Couples Relationships:

The rate of divorce and separation among parents of disabled children compared to parents of non-disabled children is a complex and varied topic. Research on this specific comparison has yielded mixed findings, and it is important to note that divorce rates can be influenced by numerous factors beyond disability alone. Partners may also sometimes feel marginalised because our children with autism require a significant amount of attention, time, and energy compared to neurotypical children. It's also fair to say that if one parent is the primary caregiver, the other partner may feel neglected, both emotionally and physically. For many men and fathers of children on the spectrum, it might manifest as a lack of physical and sexual intimacy, as they are often prioritized after their child's needs. On the other hand, mothers may feel a dearth of emotional or mental support from their husbands or partners in the daily upbringing of an autistic child. They may long for their partner to empathize with the challenges they face as caregivers and to reciprocate the understanding of how difficult it can be to raise and manage their child, particularly during the early years of diagnosis.

Several studies suggest that parents of children with disabilities may have a slightly higher divorce rate compared to parents of typically developing children. However, the differences reported in those studies were often small and not statistically significant. It is also worth noting that divorce rates in general have increased over the years, and this trend is observed across various populations. It is crucial to approach this topic with sensitivity and avoid generalizations. Each family's experience is unique, and the impact of having a disabled child on marital stability can vary widely. Seeking support, open communication, and access to appropriate resources can positively influence marital outcomes for parents of disabled children. Factors such as socioeconomic status, parental stress, available support networks, and coping mechanisms play significant roles in marital outcomes for all parents, including those with disabled children. So, it is important to consider that while raising a child with disabilities may present unique challenges, it does not necessarily determine the outcome of a marriage.

Many couples successfully navigate these challenges and maintain healthy and fulfilling relationships, while some like my own marriage do not. So, writing this chapter has been a challenging task as it brought back many complex memories and emotions that I would rather forget. However, I want to make it clear that this will not be a story of blaming my ex-wife, Pheobe. It's important to recognize that in such situations, no one truly emerges as a winner. Phoebe and I used to be happy together. We met when I was nineteen, got engaged after five months, and tied the knot when I was twenty-one. Six months later, we purchased our first home, and at the age of twenty-five, our first child, Rose, came into our lives. Five years later, our second child, Rory, was born.

Sometime around the period when Rory began exhibiting signs of being developmentally delayed compared to his peers, Phoebe and I started growing apart. As I mentioned in previous chapters, I stubbornly refused to accept that my son was different or faced any challenges. I started working more and sleeping less, gradually isolating myself from the family unit and sinking into depression. The distance between Phoebe and me widened, although neither of us could foresee it. Phoebe at that time would often express feeling like a "single mother," which was certainly due to my increased absence and the fact that when working as a postman I had been more involved in raising our children. Though it was likely to be a combination of factors.

Eventually, Phoebe and I decided to separate, and initially, it was amicable. I held myself responsible for the split, so there was no one else to blame. However, several months later, I joined an online dating site not with the intention to date, but rather as a distraction during my long work shifts, to chat with real people. That's when I met Jennifer. She sent similar detailed and scripted messages like mine, but more importantly, we connected over our children and past marriages. After two months of online conversations, we decided to meet in person.

Meeting Jennifer was a transformative experience. Her caring and maternal nature were immediately apparent, and in retrospect, it was different from what I had experienced with Phoebe. Jennifer was a successful single mother who had left her husband twice before, only returning after five years of separation when he claimed to have changed and her children desired a more united family environment. Jennifer and Phoebe couldn't have been more different in terms of independence, confidence, and personalities. As months went by, the gap between Jennifer and me narrowed, while the divide between Phoebe and me widened.

Eventually, Phoebe suspected I was involved with another woman, and it was then that Jennifer gave me an ultimatum: either start a potential new life with her or try to salvage what was left with my wife. This impromptu decision was thrust upon me when Phoebe contacted Jennifer via text, telling her to stay away from her husband. I had only a few hours to make a decision, so I turned to my best friend, Bryan, for an honest and unbiased opinion. I called him in tears while making my eventual decision. I didn't hate

Phoebe, but I no longer loved her as a husband should. It sounds clichéd, but she had become more like a sister to me for many years.

However, I didn't know any different because I had met her at a young age. We had been together since I was eighteen, and back then, we were essentially children ourselves, with little aspirations other than being seen as adults by the world. At the time, I thought that meant getting married and buying a house as soon as possible. Looking back, I don't regret anything from my past because it has shaped who I am today. However, I would advise my own children to wait until they are thirty years old, have found their calling, and established their place in the world.

Anyhow, I moved in with Jennifer, and I was a mess. I deeply missed my children, and I had caused a rift between my parents, grandparents, and extended family as they disagreed with my decision. They believed the children would be most affected by it. Some even suggested Pheobe and I remain separated but to continue to live in the same home for the sake of the children until they reached adulthood and were independent. Knowing what I know now about the likely living assistance an autistic individual requires throughout life, there's a good chance I would still be living in the same house as my now ex-wife with Rory for the rest of his life, and waiting for myself to start anew. However, I didn't choose that path. I felt happier in myself with Jen, but I also spiralled deeper into depression, burdened by guilt for abandoning my children.

Fortunately, Jen was understanding and supportive, allowing me to see the children as often as possible, which initially amounted to about three days out of seven in a week. I consider myself incredibly lucky. Jen took a considerable risk by inviting me into her home and starting a new relationship with me and her children. She has been more than I could have hoped for as a stepmother, even to this day. However, that didn't prevent me from descending further into depression as I juggled financial responsibilities with my ex-wife and the family home, built a relationship with Jen, managed the mounting costs of two households, and dealt with the rejection and estrangement from extended family members who had received a narrative of events from Phoebe that didn't always align with my own.

I continued struggling until early 2014 when anxiety started to consume me. At that point, I knew something was seriously wrong with me, so I reluctantly spoke to my doctor and completed a depression questionnaire. It's an understatement to say that I scored high as a risk. My doctor prescribed an antidepressant and sleeping tablets and assured me that things would improve within a month or two. However, my mind remained in turmoil, plagued by guilt over what I had potentially done to my family. I worried that if something happened to Jennifer and me, I would be utterly alone since my family likely wouldn't forgive me, and Phoebe had already moved on and started a new relationship, and in doing so was splitting her time and attention between her new partner and the children, and this is perhaps when Rory's behaviour really began to change for the worse, as his crisis-meltdowns, and outbursts had become far more extreme in their nature, particularly after staying with Jen and I and it was then time to return him home to his mother, this after a few months started to trouble me as I knew something had changed and wasn't right, but what. Not being part of the everyday family unit anymore meant I was mostly in the dark what with Rory being mostly non-verbal at that age, with only the occasional words making sense. The thought of burdening Jennifer with my worries and troubles weighed heavily on me because that's how I felt—a burden to her, as these were my children, my ex-partner and therefor my problems.

This went on for months and I only got worse but eventually in mid-November of 2015 it led me to a point where, after spending a weekend with the children, sorting my belongings, and saying my goodbyes through messages and texts, I found myself walking a mile or so toward a bridge on a local arterial road. I sat on the edge of the bridge, contemplating jumping and relieving the burdens on those around me. In that state of mind, I didn't believe suicide was a selfish act; in fact, it felt like the opposite. I thought I was lightening the worry and burden I imposed on my loved ones. Yes, I wanted to feel better, which is why I sought help and started taking antidepressants. But there I was, on the verge of *a "permanent solution to a temporary problem,"* as the late comedian and fellow depression sufferer Robin Williams once said.

As I sat, watching the traffic flow beneath me, I reflected on the last moments I might ever have and remembered the last book I had read to Rory only hours earlier, "Peppa Pig's My Daddy." The book's final sentence went something like, "My daddy is the best daddy in the whole world." In that moment, I wondered who would understand and be patient enough with Rory when I was gone. Who would protect and teach him better than me? The answer was no one. No one could be me for Rory, no matter how hard they tried or succeeded, because he would always know the difference. Despite his autism, Rory has a remarkable memory.

I stood up from the bridge and embarked on the shameful journey back to the apartment, sniffling and sobbing the entire way. What I had done seemed like a cry for attention, to some extent, but it didn't feel that way at the time. I wanted to die, but I didn't want to be the one to make that decision and never see my son and daughter again. I wanted someone else to take my life, but of course, that wasn't likely to happen within the thirty minutes it took to walk home. When I arrived, the police, my best friend Bryan, and Jen were waiting for me. I sat down and cried, confessing what I had intended to do and why. One of the police officers, a man, said something that still resonates with me today: "Six months ago, I was in the same place as you, and I promise you can overcome this. You will get better."

I'm not sure if it was because Jen, dressed in her full paramedic uniform, having left work to get to me or because I was brutally honest with everyone, but the police didn't detain me under the Mental Health Act. I promised everyone, right then and there, that I would seek immediate help, and I believe I spent the rest of the day in bed, exhausted from the previous sleepless night spent planning my suicide. I cried myself to sleep, and when sleep finally took me, I was ready.

The following day, and true to my word, Jen and I contacted my employer, explaining what had happened and requesting some time off. I couldn't help but feel guilty about it, knowing that finding replacements for our roles for the facility I worked in at the time wouldn't be easy for my manager. However, he proved to be empathetic and understanding. Then came the moment I had been avoiding—the hospital visit. I had been trying to come up with excuses to avoid it, including the call to work. As I entered the mental health unit of the hospital, it felt like entering a low-security prison. I sat in the waiting area, secretly considering escape plans in case they decided to detain me against my will. I eventually met a mental health doctor and nurse, who discussed my issues and recent life choices at length, and then debated over medication and a possible way forward for me. Recounting what I'd almost done the day prior again sent me into a maelstrom of emotions ranging from guilt, gratitude, and shame, but also love.

The next month or so was trying, the specialists referred me to a crisis team with a 24hr telephone number to discuss anything negative above if I needed it, they also made occasional home visits early on, but to be honest the medication they put me on was the most spaced out I've ever been in my life, so pretty much prevented me from doing anything mentally challenging, let alone physically. I spent an early part of my recovery just sleeping, which was definitely a medicine that my body and mind really needed. After a few weeks the new anti-depressants I was prescribed started to take effect and I became more relaxed and was able to think with better clarity about day-to-day things rather than obsesses or worry about things I had little to no control over like Jen being attacked or having an accident in her job. I was before always worrying about things, thinking the worst about things that may never happen, but yet would play scenarios out in my head and then obsess about them and that's when I'd become anxious and unable to sleep., but now those thoughts were subsiding and I was able to look for other things to distract me and be able to return to work. This was now February of 2016, a new year and a new start, but I still wasn't a hundred percent back to being myself, and I still had Rory who's outbursts and behaviour had become so regular, yet unpredictable that he was excluded permanently from his special needs school, so the worries started to bubble up again and I was given a higher dosage of anti-depressant to help stay at the level of objective mental clarity that I'd recently re-acquired.

This is when I sort further distractions in the way of academic research and combining my love of the natural world and wildlife, but also in getting a dog, which we weren't allowed at the apartment, but we managed to find a work around, and not one I'm proud to have undertook but it served its purpose and ultimately worked out for the benefit of all the family. Dogs will always enjoy a walk and regardless of your mood whether that be high or low, they will want to pay you attention and will love you unconditionally regardless of their age. So, Zorro our new family addition provided a lot of mental and physical distraction in his training and socialisation and in a way filled a gap I was missing in the daily absence of my children. Then there was the Open University Open Access course, which for anyone that failed in education, as I pretty much had. It meant I could take a module that tested my English, Math, and Science skills some twenty years after I'd left secondary school. It was only a six-month course and I managed to pass it with a distinction and that encouraged me to pursue my interest in a particular career I'd always dreamed of having which was to become a national park ranger in the Welsh valleys or perhaps the Highlands, but to achieve this I first needed a degree in environmental management. I can honestly say that between the Open University stimulating my mind and distracting me with its degree content, it helped steer some of the less positive thoughts into neutral and academic and thoughts instead. After the first year of study, I switched to a science degree instead, due to another life change and one that was to influence my children's, ex-wife and new families lives to this day in a mostly positive manner.

In 2017, concerns arose from Rory's school and social care about the challenges my ex-wife, Pheobe, was facing in raising Rory. She was navigating the complexities of a new relationship and co-parenting our children, a task I understood to be difficult even without the additional challenges of caring for an autistic child like Rory. During this period, our co-parenting relationship hit its lowest point, marked by frequent disagreements, harsh words, and differences in parenting approaches for our children, though especially Rory.

As the pressure of juggling multiple responsibilities became overwhelming for Pheobe, local agencies intervened, and Jennifer and I stepped in to take on the daily care of the children. Eventually, we had to move back to the family home to provide a stable environment for the children and their educations, while Pheobe relocated nearby to offer her continued support while settling into a new home with her current partner, Phil, with whom she still resides.

Over time, wounds on both sides have healed, and we have managed to develop a more amicable and communicative co-parenting relationship, primarily centred around the welfare of our children. Today, we work together to ensure that Rory and Rose receive the love, care, and support they need, embracing the challenges of parenthood as a united front.

Relationships with our other children:

At the time before Rory's birth, I wasn't particularly enthusiastic about having another child, but I can't say I was coerced into it. Phoebe simply didn't want our daughter to grow up as an only child, just like she had. On the other hand, I was content with the idea of Rose being the perfect little person we had already brought into this world. I also had concerns about not being able to feel the same love for another child as I felt for Rose. However, my mother, who had raised me and my younger brother, reassured me that I would love them both equally, albeit in different ways. Looking back now, over a decade later, my mother was right. Both children are unique individuals, and I do love them both equally. However, those who have a differently abled or disabled child, like Rory, understand that we tend to give more attention to that child. Like me, they may often feel as if they are neglecting their more capable older child, Rose, by not always providing her with equal time and attention.

Some years later in 2018 I found myself sitting outside St. Botolph Church near Aldgate Station in London. I am here with Rose. As she's grown older, our time together diminishes, so even if it's just accompanying her to places, it's a chance to catch up without the distractions of home life. I am writing this while sitting outside the church on a lovely sunny day in April. I could have chosen to walk ten minutes down the road and sip on Starbucks for three hours, but I decided to stay close during this bank holiday weekend Saturday because I am sometimes overly concerned about security and safety. From where I'm sitting, I have a direct view of the main entrance of the building, which gives me peace of mind knowing Rose is safe inside. The same goes for her when she steps onto the street; she knows my location as we circled the building before finding my preferred vantage point. Planning is part of my character and lifestyle now, as most outings have become planned and rehearsed due to Rory's autism.

I love my daughter immensely, and she is one of the most confident individuals I know, sometimes even speaking her mind too freely. However, she is still learning, as am I but I hope she becomes a very independent individual who succeeds in whatever path she chooses. Her relationship with her brother has been and still is fairly good, though due to the five-year age gap they have little in common, but they are both generally always polite and courteous towards one another. Rose will still take the occasional whack, or have her hair pulled by Rory when he's distressed, but thankfully these have gotten less frequent as they have both developed into teenagers and for Rose as a young adult. Rose and I have however talked about Rory always needing a little more assistance and attention than your average child such as herself, regardless of this she would on rare occasions say I was favouring Rory over her or letting him get away with something, which nearly always wasn't true, but it doesn't stop the sting of such comments from your own child making you feel guilty as a parent. This I remind myself is typical behaviour for any child to use such phrases against their parent's decisions, even if that decision is justified and warranted.

My position at the church is on a bench to the side, adjacent to two homeless individuals named Kevin and his new friend, Peter. Peter has an American accent but was originally born in Manchester and presumably returned there later in his life. Kevin, who is forty-two, and Peter, who is in his eighties, struck up a conversation when Kevin commented on the weather. Overhearing their interaction, it is evident that these gentlemen, despite their circumstances, behave with courtesy and respect in each other's company. They are true gentlemen.

It's interesting to note that no one else in the vicinity seems to acknowledge or make eye contact with them. In fact, one woman even sneered as she walked past while Peter was removing his socks to air his feet. This act made me chuckle as Rory won't wear socks or shoes given the choice, and at the first opportunity, he will remove them if they aren't necessary.

Now in 2023, I have learned, to make time for both of my children, though in truth, it hasn't been in equal measure, but when does it ever? When any second or successive children are born, the need for care and attention for that child is always going to be greater than for the one beforehand. The bigger the age gaps between the children, the more independent the first child is going to be. So, now Rory is fourteen and Rose is nineteen. Rose rarely comes to me for companionship or escorting to social events or to friends' homes anymore. Instead, she comes to me when she needs help with academic advice, my point of view, or the age-old request "Can I borrow some money?"—borrow meaning can I have and not pay back the money!

Rory too has developed, not to the extent that a typical boy his age would, but it's development, nevertheless. He can now run a bath and bathe himself, make a drink, toast with butter and marmite, and can take himself to the toilet. He now understands the need to wash clothing and change bedding, but without being prompted of such necessities and reminded of them, it does mean that for now, he'll likely never live a fully independent life and will always need some form of assistance. How much of his life will require assisted living in the future remains, for now, unknown, but the next decade should give an indication and will probably be in another book chronicling the challenges of our relationship together as he transitions into adulthood.

Extended Family Relationships:

A recent study (Bessette Gorlin, 2016) explored the experiences of families raising children with severe autism and/or comorbidity conditions, including extended family members and friends. Surprisingly, many families developed "hybrid or blended families" that blurred the lines between nuclear and extended family, showing how various relatives and friends contributed to caregiving and emotional support. Grandparents, particularly grandmothers, played crucial roles in assisting parents with cooking, cleaning, and caring for the child, allowing parents to take breaks. Some grandparents took on long-term planning for the child's future care. Extended family members emphasized the unique and intimate care they provided, differentiating it from external support. Families also shared the challenges of navigating public perceptions and stereotypes about autism, often facing stigma, humiliation, and isolation due to their child's behaviours in public places. Unfortunately, as my parents had me so young themselves, they still haven't reached retirement age and thus their time was often limited in offering support through childcare or respite.

Relationships with social friends and/or work colleagues:

From the same 2016 study, many families felt misunderstood and wished for more understanding and support from the public, highlighting the need for better awareness of autism's invisible nature. Academic settings were also a source of isolation and conflict for some families, with children not fully integrated into the classroom, and confrontations leading to some children being removed from settings. Overall, the study shed light on the complexities and support networks within families raising autistic children, while also emphasizing the need for greater societal understanding and inclusion.

Having firsthand experience of isolation as both a child and parent in group gatherings can be painful and isolating, especially when Rory's peers excluded him from birthday parties due to his previous outbursts. While I understand parents wanting to safeguard their children, if I didn't have a broader understanding of autism, I might have done the same.

The challenges started to emerge when Rory's behaviour affected his health and that of his nursery peers, leading to early pick-ups from the nursery. At that time, we hadn't yet started questioning or pursuing a diagnosis, and not knowing about his different needs caused additional stress. This led to work-related issues, with me being labelled awkward, and ultimately losing my job due to my poor choices and lack of communication. Looking back, I now realize that it was the beginning of my journey into depression.

Nowadays, I am open about our challenges, centred around Rory's routine and care, but during those pre-diagnosis years, it was rough on our family, friends, and work colleagues, and for that, I apologize for the poor choices I sometimes made back then.

Although times are changing, some men may still feel solely responsible as the primary wage earners, expecting their wives to primarily handle the responsibilities of children and domestic chores within the family unit. This perspective may persist, regardless of whether the wife works part-time or full-time, which is increasingly common in today's modern society. However, whether the wife works or not is generally irrelevant. Both our relationships with our partners and our children can only benefit from a more equitable distribution of responsibilities.

Chapter VIII

Relationships Part 2

"All that I am, or hope to be, I owe to my mother" - Abraham Lincoln

In the intricate tapestry of modern families, there exists a profound and undeniable truth: that for most of us, the well-being of our children is paramount. Amid the complexities of separated or divorced parents, step-parents, and new partners, one fundamental principle emerges—a united front is essential for the betterment of any child. For that very reason, it is important that I also give others close to Rory a chance to say a little about their experience, challenges, and life's journey they have shared.

This chapter delves into the significance of these diverse family roles, driven by a shared dedication to nurturing, guiding, and fostering an environment where Rory could flourish. Here, I hope to explore the extraordinary potential that emerges when adults put aside differences, ego, and past grievances, and focus their energies on what truly matters—the happiness and growth of their children. Drawing on stories and experiences, both Rory's mother and stepmother give their narratives to this chapter and the benefits that arise when separated or divorced parents, step-parents, and partners work together.

Through the lens of these blended families, I hope to instil how mutual respect and cooperation can offer our autistic children a stable foundation in an ever-changing world. As we journey through this chapter, we'll discover that it is not only possible but imperative that adults, no matter their roles or histories, unite for the greater good—creating an enduring legacy of love, support, and shared responsibility.

Pheobe: Rory's Mum

Hi, I'm Pheobe

Rory's mother and I first became aware of Rory's differences when the nursery he attended pulled my husband Matt and me aside to discuss his behaviours. They believed he might have Autism. Initially, I wondered how they arrived at that conclusion based on his behaviour alone. However, it became clear that there were other reasons, such as his slow development, that led them to this assessment.

One of the most memorable challenges I faced with Rory was when he would have meltdowns in the middle of a supermarket or other public places. I couldn't pick him up to comfort him because I wasn't strong enough to do so without risking being kicked or having my hair pulled. The stares and comments from strangers made me feel like a bad mother, as they didn't understand that his meltdowns were a result of his Autism, not his misbehaviour.

Rory now lives with his dad Matt, stepmom Jen, and our daughter Rose, but I see him every weekend and some weekdays during school holidays. This routine was put in place to cater to his specific needs. Initially, he struggled to adapt to it and would become very anxious. However, over time, he has become more comfortable when I visit, he's very chatty, asking about my breakfast and sharing in simple joys.

My work with adults with learning disabilities has given me insights into traits similar to my son Rory's. They often exhibit repetitive speech, struggle with eye contact, display challenging behaviours, and experience meltdowns. Yet, they are also incredibly caring and empathetic, just like Rory.

Over the years, my relationship with Rory had its ups and downs, especially during his meltdowns. He was once very cuddly and content living with me, but then he started having meltdowns at home a lot more with me. It seemed like he was calmer with his dad and Jen, and I felt hurt and disconnected for a while. However, as time passed, he became more at ease when he knew I was coming to see him, and our bond rekindled.

As Rory's mother, I support his choices within the community and his family life. He will always need support, and I'll be there for him through life changes and any challenges he may face. Even when he eventually moves away with his dad and Jen, I'll continue to visit and help him with life skills.

When Rory received a "Star of the Week" award from his teacher for his excellent performance in class, I was proud of him, even though I knew that too much attention stressed him out. He understood my pride without me having to express it overtly.

Initially, when Rory was diagnosed with Autism, I didn't fully comprehend what it meant. However, now working with adults with learning disabilities who also had Autism and participating in an Autism bus workshop provided me with a deeper understanding and empathy. I learned the importance of giving individuals with Autism time, patience, and space during difficult moments.

To other parents with autistic children, I would say that you'll have both good and challenging days. Be patient and understanding and try to empathize with their feelings. It's also crucial to include siblings, as I regret that my daughter Rose sometimes felt left out due to Rory's meltdowns. As she grew up, she developed a deep understanding of her brother's condition and became incredibly supportive.

My personal growth and character development have given me insight into the challenges faced by people with Autism, allowing me to understand their reactions better.

One of the most pleasant surprises has been witnessing Rory's progress in school. His speech has improved significantly, and he's become calmer during car rides, no longer unbuckling his seatbelt, or throwing things out the window. Despite changes in teachers, Rory has adapted well. I'm immensely proud of the funny and loving young man he's becoming, knowing that he will always have challenges but also the unwavering love and support of our family.

I will forever be a part of Rory's life. Even as he leaves school and moves on, I'll be there to offer support and help with any challenges he encounters. With the love and support of his dad, sister, stepmom, and our extended family, Rory will always have a network of people who cherish him and stand by him through life's struggles and triumphs as he grows into the remarkable young man he's becoming.

Jennifer: Rory's Step-Mum

Hi, I'm Jen,

A Little About Me.

Before I met Matt in 2013, I was a divorced, single mother of three children: Emily, my eldest, and two boys, George, the middle child, and Apollo, the youngest. I'd been a single mother for a few years due to the breakdown of my first marriage and had to move out of the family home with my children. The four of us now lived in a three-bedroom flat. I was completing a university course in emergency medicine and working full-time in the emergency services. Emily was at college and working, and Apollo, the youngest, was still in full-time education, pursuing A-levels and planning on attending university. Meanwhile, George was at college and planning on going to university also. All three of my children had gone through mainstream primary and secondary schools. Despite some instances of bullying, they managed well and moved on to college.

When my children were born, I wanted to be a stay-at-home mom because I believed it was crucial to be with them during their early years, before they started primary school. I had three children under the age of 3, with my daughter Emily at 2 and a half, and George at 1 and a half when I had Apollo. My time as a full-time mom involved managing the household, taking my children to parks and playgroups, appointments and check-ups, shopping, trips out, reading books and playing games, cooking, and housework. My daily routine revolved around my children. I regularly took my children on holidays to Devon to see their great nan while their father worked full-time as a salesman. I joined the National Childbirth Trust and volunteered to help with the playgroups they organized. Once, my youngest, Apollo started primary school, I became a teaching assistant to align my working hours with their school hours.

For the next eight years, I worked as a full-time teaching assistant, supporting children with additional needs in mainstream schools. These children had various challenges, including physical and sensory impairments, learning disabilities, autism, Asperger's syndrome, or other emotional and behavioural difficulties. My role involved helping these children with their education and social development.

When my youngest child started secondary school and could manage his own morning routine, I decided it was time for a career change. In my younger years, I had an interest in the army, having been a member of the army cadets and adventure scouts, prior to that brownies and guides. I loved hiking, camping, and sports, even representing my school in swimming, running, and athletics, including javelin.

I reached a point in my life where I was regaining my freedom and wanted to try something new. So, I applied to the NHS for a job in the emergency services, which involved working 12-hour shifts, both day and night, while also studying for a university qualification in emergency medicine. I got the job, which I still love and have been doing for over 15 years now.

Towards the end of my training, I started talking to Matt. I came across a picture of him holding his two-year-old son before I physically met him. The photo captured a genuine moment of love between a father and his child, Matt smiling at his son and his son smiling back with the most genuine smile a happy child could give. This told me everything I needed to know about Matt—he loved his children.

When I finally met Matt's children, Rory was three and undergoing assessments at the local child development assessment clinic. I was familiar with the clinic because I had taken my own son, George, there when he was in primary school due to behavioural changes. George was diagnosed with speech and language difficulties and social communication disorder. He underwent speech and language therapy and was able to remain in his class, performing at the same level as his peers in mainstream education. His behaviour improved once he received this diagnosis, and his teacher adapted his approach to teaching him, leading to a positive outcome for everyone.

I noticed that Rory, at three years old, exhibited slightly different behaviour than my own children did at that age. However, I attributed it to his young age and figured he might be experiencing a slight delay in speech development, much like my son Apollo, who didn't start speaking until he was two years old. Matt took Rory to his assessments and was deeply involved in his children's care.

75

When I first met Rose, she was eight years old and leading a normal, happy life in mainstream primary school. Rose possessed a remarkable singing talent and attended acting and singing classes, as well as scouts. I vividly remember attending her school plays with Matt, where she outshone everyone with her singing. We attended Rose's sports events and took the children on camping holidays to Devon, which Rory particularly enjoyed. They stayed with us in my flat when Matt had rest days from work, which amounted to three to four days a week.

When Rory was diagnosed with autism and developmental delay following multiple assessments at the clinic, he was four years old. Having worked with children with autism before, I wasn't particularly fazed by the diagnosis. In my eyes, I loved Matt, their father, and the children came with him, much like my own children came with me. Although, my children were much older now— Apollo was heading to university, Emily had moved into her own flat, and George was relocating to Cornwall—I was an experienced mother and felt at ease with Matt having younger children.

During this period, Matt was working full-time in security, and the children, Rory, and Rose, were living with their mother in the family home they had always known. They stayed with us three to four days/nights a week and were always happy to stay and seemed to settle with us quickly. However, it became increasingly challenging to return Rory to his mother. He would often protest, experience meltdowns, scream, hit, and pull hair, refusing to walk to her car, or even leave the flat, if we told him where he was going. Phoebe, his mother, endured more of these outbursts when Rory was at home with her, where he would hit her, pull her hair, throw objects like shoes, toys, and even his iPads over the garden fence or out of the car window. He would also pull on the TV wiring and TV channel boxes, frequently breaking them. Additionally, he would throw his mother's mobile phone into the toilet or clog the toilet with clothing or toys causing a flood.

76

Matt was constantly worried about his children during this period and concerned about Phoebe's well-being at home due to Rory's challenging behaviour. Phoebe kept requesting Matt and me to have the children more frequently. Rory often arrived at our place without spare clothes, shoes, or toys. I transitioned back into a maternal role and bought Rory clothes, shoes, and toys, all of which stayed at the flat. I wanted Rory to feel as comfortable as possible with us, as I understood that disruptions to routines could upset him. Consequently, I accommodated his needs.

Under the weight of his concerns for his children when they weren't with us, Matt's mental health began to deteriorate. It was heart-wrenching to see Rory's distress when leaving us to return home to his mother. Matt fell into depression, and I observed a change in his behaviour. Matt reached a point where he had to take a break from work to focus on improving his mental health, receiving the necessary support. After some time, Matt was able to return to work, and his mental health gradually improved. Social support was also implemented for Phoebe at home with Rory. However, there remained a stark contrast in Rory's behaviour between our home and his mother's.

Rory was calmer and exhibited fewer behavioural issues while staying with us. Social services monitored his behaviour at home with Phoebe and noticed that Rory seemed more agitated and anxious there, leading to more frequent and severe behavioural problems. We needed to pay close attention to Rory's behaviour in various environments and identify factors that triggered his anxiety or contributed to its alleviation. Social services observed Rory interacting with Matt and me at our flat and noted that he was much calmer there.

Although Rory has severe autism and developmental delay, he could express his preferences about where he wanted to stay, and his behaviour indicated his anxiety levels in various environments. Rory started living with us full-time, and we no longer required social services' intervention in his care. Eventually, his sister Rose also began living with us full-time six months later. With both Rory and Rose staying with us full-time, Matt left full-time work and took on the role of a full-time carer for Rory and Rose, working part-time around the needs and routine of the children who were 8 and 13 at this point.

My initial impression of Rory was that he understood more than he could verbally express. Rory always seemed to be listening to us, even when he was playing on his iPad or with his toys or puzzles. If when talking Matt or me said something he didn't like his behaviour would change from happily playing to hitting or throwing his iPad or books. We needed to be careful what and who we were discussing around him as he understood, even though he couldn't verbalise, his change in body language spoke volumes.

To ensure his comfort and reduce the risk of meltdowns, I adopted a daily routine and explained everything we were doing or planning to do. This preparation was crucial for outings and park visits. When Rory went swimming with us for the first time, I recall Matt mentioning that they had attempted it before, but Rory didn't enjoy it, so they hadn't gone again. I wanted to give it a try to understand why he didn't like it and, if possible, help him develop a liking for swimming—a skill I believed was essential for children to learn.

On the day of our swimming trip, we informed Rory in advance, and he didn't protest, which is a positive start. We drove to the swimming pool. Rory came with us willingly, entered the changing rooms, got changed without a fuss, and then we headed to the pool area. As we approached the poolside, Rory hesitated and began to display signs of anxiety and agitation. Matt picked him up and took him straight into the water, where Rory became increasingly distressed. I suggested to Matt, that Rory and I sit together on the poolside for a moment before entering the water and Matt take Rose in the pool. I sensed that Rory was becoming overstimulated by the noise and the presence of other people in the echoing pool area. My hope was that sitting on the bench area for a while, in view of the pool, would allow him to adjust, observe, and understand his surroundings better, thereby reducing his anxiety.

Rory sat with me, and together, we watched the people in the family pool, splashing and playing around. It didn't take long for Rory to calm down, and he even began to smile at the people having fun. Once I felt he was ready, I asked if we could move to the steps in the shallow end of the pool, just to dip our feet in. Rory agreed, and we sat on the steps, playfully splashing our feet, which made him laugh. It soon became evident that Rory enjoyed splashing the water, especially if he could target me or his dad. He ventured further into the pool, and we had fun splashing each other while his dad would disappear under the water and tickle his feet. We had successfully introduced Rory to the pool and made many more swimming trips after this. He'd head straight for the steps to splash his feet before eventually submerging himself, if his feet could touch the pool floor, he revelled in swimming and splashing around.

I found that maintaining a daily routine and explaining everything to Rory helped keep his anxiety levels in check, preventing meltdowns. Every child is unique, but I believe most if not all children benefit from routines, advance preparation for changes, and explanations when facing new experiences. They need time to adapt to new environments to feel comfortable and at ease.

As a couple, Matt and I believe we parent Rory effectively. When I first met Rory, my prior experience as a mother of three children allowed me to easily adapt to the role of a stepmother. My primary objective was to make Rory feel comfortable around me, ensuring that he was happy and relaxed during his stays with us. We established a stable routine that reduced his anxiety levels, introduced new activities after thorough explanations, and maintained open communication. Rory had his own room filled with toys, puzzles, books, and sensory lights, creating a calming and safe space for him.

We together attended family gatherings, birthday celebrations, and dined at restaurants with Rory's grandparents frequently. We participated in his school events, maintaining regular communication with the school to understand his progress and interactions with other children. I like to think that we functioned well as a team, serving as good role models for Rory. It's crucial for children to witness positive interactions between their caregivers, and we are mindful of the language we use when referring to each other. Rory started calling us "his parents," although I understand that it can occasionally cause confusion for those working with him at school. It's essential to distinguish between me as "Mum Jen" and his biological mother as "Mum Phoebe" to prevent Rory from becoming distressed.

Every child is different and develops at their own pace, although this is influenced by their environment and various other factors like family structure, different child rearing methods, also providing a healthy diet, where they feel safe and can grow up in a healthy atmosphere with the freedom to express themselves. They each possess their individual personalities within the family unit and form connections with people in their lives. I'm grateful to be a part of Rory's life and to have the opportunity to influence and support him emotionally and mentally during a challenging period.

Raising a child, especially one with disabilities, can be challenging for any family. Balancing the roles of parent, caregiver, employee, and self-care can be difficult. Parents often neglect their own needs, unable to find time for personal pursuits. During my earlier years as a mother of three small children, my days revolved around their care and were filled with various daily tasks, from morning routines through to bedtime.

As a parent or caregiver, it's easy to lose one's identity as individual needs are placed on hold indefinitely. Parenting is a full-time responsibility, and ensuring that children receive the best nurturing, safe, and supportive environment is paramount. Meeting their physical, emotional, and mental needs is essential. Children need emotional support, mental stimulation, care during illness, comfort during distress, and guidance in making good choices and forming healthy relationships. They require a nurturing environment, routine, consistency, understanding, patience, and encouragement.

Children also learn from observing their parents and caregivers, so positive interactions and role modelling are crucial. Clear communication and shared responsibilities between partners are vital to avoid resentment and maintain a healthy family dynamic. Making time for each other as a couple is equally important, as it allows for relaxation and quality time away from parenting responsibilities.

Ultimately, the reward of seeing a child grow into a healthy, independent, confident, and happy adult makes all the challenges and sacrifices worthwhile.

I hope that my older children feel that I did my best for them, and I aspire to provide the same level of care and support for Rory and his sister as a stepmother as they grow into adulthood.

Chapter IX

Autism Media Portrayals

"May I say that I have not thoroughly enjoyed serving with Humans?

I find their illogic and foolish emotions a constant irritant".

- Mr Spock, Star Trek

If you're a fan of either of the two recent television shows that debuted globally "Atypical" on the streaming service Netflix or "The Good Doctor" on ABC — I've got news for you. You're watching an overly positive depiction of autism that doesn't reflect reality for the majority of people on the spectrum or their families.

To the TV-watching public, autism has generally come to mean the verbal, higher-skilled, savant end of the spectrum because individuals at that end make for interesting characters.

In "Atypical," the protagonist Sam's autism complicates the typical struggles high school students face, from finding a girlfriend to fitting in with the popular teens. But Sam never seems to spend any time in a special education classroom, much less at a special school.

In "The Good Doctor," Shaun, the eponymous doctor, struggles with the stress of being a brilliant surgeon. He's a compelling character but a far cry from most nonverbal, intellectually disabled adults with autism who struggle to find any job at all.

And in "The Big Bang Theory," a wildly popular comedy that has been on the air for 10 years, one of the leading characters, Sheldon, is a scientific genius with Asperger syndrome-like tendencies. But unlike many adults with autism, Sheldon lives with his friends. His habit of knocking three times on his neighbour Penny's door is seen as cute and endearing.

Based on my past experiences, most adult men around my age, of forty-five, who are unfamiliar with the world of autism don't know much about the subject besides what they have seen portrayed in the media. If there're lucky, they may have watched or at least heard of the movie "Rain Man," starring Dustin Hoffman as the autistic brother Raymond Babbitt and Tom Cruise as his neurotypical younger sibling Charles. If you then start to explain, "Yes, like Rain Man, but he's a savant, and there are inconsistencies in the movie regarding some of his autistic traits," your average man at this point will likely just zone out and change the subject, not knowing what the heck you are talking about.

The movie actually drew inspiration from an individual named Kim Peek, whom I guarantee virtually no one has ever heard of. Kim was born with brain damage. A doctor later told Kim's father, Francis, that Kim's severe developmental disabilities would not allow him to walk, let alone learn anything significant. The doctor's prognosis was to have Kim institutionalized and forget about the boy. Thankfully, Kim's father disregarded the doctor's advice.

Throughout his life, Kim struggled with typical motor skills and had difficulty walking. He was considered severely disabled, couldn't button his shirts, and tested below average on general IQ tests. However, for all that Kim lacked in one area of his life, he made up for it in almost inconceivable ways in others. During his lifetime, Kim had read around 12,000 books and could remember almost everything about their content. Consider that against the most recent Kindle from Amazon, which can hold perhaps say 1,100 books out of the box. Kim could read two pages at once, with his left eye reading the left page and his right eye reading the right page. It would take him approximately 3 seconds to read through two pages. Kim could recall facts and figures from multiple subject areas, ranging from geography and history to sports. When given a date, Kim was able to tell you what day of the week it was. He was also able to remember every piece of music he had ever heard. He was a remarkable individual yet needed assisted living support throughout his life, often provided by his father.

Kim sadly passed away in December 2009 at the age of 58, as the result of a heart attack. Since then, there has been some question as to the accuracy of Kim's original diagnosis of autism. Personally, I'd like to think that whatever Kim's disability was, it was secondary to his talents and the challenges that many disabled individuals must overcome in a world geared towards able-bodied and neurotypical individuals.

If it weren't for Kim and the love and support of his father, we wouldn't have had the inspiration for "Rain Man" and while that movie is fine as a form of entertainment, it does little to enlighten the average viewer about the challenges faced by parents, children, or even autistic adults in their everyday lives, with or without savant qualities. For those starting their autism journey of discovery and who are not familiar with the term "savant," a savant is often defined as a person with a developmental disorder, such as autism, who exhibits exceptional skills, usually but not limited to a specialized subject like mathematics (as in Rain Man's case), art, or music. It has been estimated that approximately one in ten autistic individuals may have savant skills.

Moreover, the "Rain Man" savant stereotype creates unrealistic expectations for individuals with autism and their families. When a child with autism fails to demonstrate prodigious skills in a particular field, it can lead to disappointment or frustration from those who held such expectations. It is essential to recognize that individuals with autism, like everyone else, have their own unique strengths and challenges that extend beyond their diagnosis. Their talents and abilities should not necessarily be tied to a specific set of expectations.

More recent, film and television productions seem to have jumped on the autistic bandwagon, while the topic of autism is prominent in the public's mind, possibly due to the increase in global diagnoses. I recently watched the movie "The Predator" (2018), which is a continuation of the 1987 film "Predator" starring Arnold Schwarzenegger. In this new sequel, a child is portrayed as having autistic otherworldly abilities that could unlock the alien technology of the predators. The overarching message in this movie was that the autistic child's ability was due to his autism being an evolutionary human attribute, and this boy was akin to a superhero at the end of the movie.

Similarly, the 2017 reboot movie "Power Rangers" also featured an autistic ranger and portrayed this character as another superhero due to his abilities. I do like the idea of introducing characters with different abilities and conditions within the realm of media aimed at children to subtly educate them about the conditions of human differences, though this isn't a new concept, as shows like Star Trek in 1966 attempted the same by introducing different ethnicities, interracial relations, and even alien races.

Over the past decade, there have been a number of shows and movies introducing or featuring central or supporting characters on the autistic spectrum. While almost all serve to raise awareness of the condition, which is a good thing, the majority of these shows portray high-functioning (often savant) characters. As my academically high-functioning stepson Apollo observed, practically all the characters have all the stereotypical archetypes associated with autism thrown at them on screen. With characters often portrayed as obsessive, repetitive, socially awkward geniuses/savants who take things just a bit too literally. While these conditions are often present in some cases of autism, they differ in degree and the exhibited behaviours can manifest in different ways, because everyone is different. As the saying goes, "If you know one individual with autism, then you know one individual with autism," highlighting that we are all individuals first and foremost, and the term "autism" is second and really nothing more than a label.

We tend to label people based on different aspects, including religion, ethnicity, and of course, abilities. Most of Hollywood's autistic characters are, for the most part, just caricatures exaggerating the most prominent traits associated with the condition.

Another stereotype depicted in film and media portrays individuals with autism as violent or dangerous. This portrayal is not only inaccurate but also stigmatizing and harmful. Research does not support the notion that autistic individuals are more prone to violence than those without autism. In reality, individuals with autism are more likely to be victims of violence than perpetrators. Perpetuating this stereotype contributes to fear, mistrust, and discrimination towards individuals with the condition. It is crucial to understand that autism itself does not make someone inherently dangerous, and any violent behaviour is more likely influenced by individual factors or environmental circumstances.

From my own perspective, there is one character in pop culture media that I have often thought embodies many qualities and challenges associated with a person on the spectrum, and that character, as you might have guessed from the epigraph quote accompanying this chapter, is Mr. Spock from the TV and movie franchise Star Trek. Spock exhibits several traits and characteristics that parallel those often associated with Autism. His logical and analytical nature, combined with his struggle to understand and express human emotions, might resonate with the experiences of individuals on the autism spectrum. Like many autistic individuals, Mr. Spock often struggles with social interactions, relying on a strict adherence to logic and facts rather than intuitive or emotional cues.

His difficulty in grasping sarcasm or figurative language, along with his preference for routine and predictability, further aligns with the traits commonly seen in individuals on the spectrum. While Mr. Spock is a fictional character, his portrayal perhaps provides a more relatable representation that can help foster understanding and empathy for those on the spectrum. Also, though Mr. Spock is only half-human in the universe and time depicted in Star Trek, he benefits from a universal translator that can decipher different languages, whether they are human or alien in nature. Unfortunately, in the present real world, one clinical hallmark of autism is a lack of speech and language during childhood, with a moderate percentage of individuals with autism being nonverbal. Estimates suggest that approximately 25% to 30% of individuals with the condition may be nonverbal or like Rory have only limited speech abilities.

So, imagine the frustration you would feel if you were unable to articulate your thoughts in spoken words. People might assume that your inability to verbalize stems from lower intelligence. This problem affects individuals with autism, and I'm sure it would also have affected Mr. Spock if it were not for those marvellous universal translators.

As the stigma associated with mental disabilities begins to lift, autobiographies and films have begun to emerge. Temple Grandin, diagnosed in 1949, wrote the book "Thinking in Pictures: My Life with Autism." Then, in 2010, HBO Films produced the movie "Temple Grandin – Thinking in Pictures" starring Claire Danes. Even though Temple Grandin could not speak until the age of four and was recommended to be institutionalized, she went on to earn her Ph.D., design livestock-holding facilities that improve the conditions of animals and wrote several books. Her autobiography offers readers a glimpse into the mind of an autistic person. Most people depend on spoken and written language to communicate and are verbal thinkers, but Grandin thinks in pictures. She describes her mind as a video recorder. After mentally recording a moment or object, she can go back and see it from different angles to create novel images by combining those different viewpoints. Because Grandin thinks using free association, her mind jumps from image to image.

Even though the directors of "Temple Grandin" and "Rain Man" take creative liberties to create drama and increase viewership, these movies have increased social awareness. Ultimately, "Thinking in Pictures" is an inspirational and informative story that best illuminates the public about people who differ from the norm.

In truth, just like Mr. Spock, individuals with autism experience a wide range of emotions and are fully capable of forming strong emotional connections with their loved ones. However, their often-unique communication styles and social behaviour may differ from societal norms, making it challenging for them to express their emotions in expected ways. The stereotype of a lack of emotional connection or empathy falsely assumes that individuals with autism are unable to forge deep connections or contribute meaningfully to society. I know this firsthand as a father to a teenager on the spectrum, and I can confidently say that it is untrue. Portraying them as either savants, incapable individuals or unemotional overlooks the nuanced reality and undermines a comprehensive understanding of their abilities and feelings.

So, while there have been recent positive examples of film and media representations of autism, there is still much progress to be made in accurately and authentically portraying autism in media. It is essential for media creators and producers to collaborate with autistic individuals to ensure their perspectives and experiences are faithfully represented on screen. As many individuals with the condition actively work to promote understanding and acceptance and I'm happy to say there has been a positive shift since starting this book with docu-films like:

"Autism in Love" (2015):

This film explores the experiences of four people on the autism spectrum as they navigate the complexities of romantic relationships.

"Neurotypical" (2013):

This documentary provides a diverse perspective on autism by interviewing people with the condition, their families, and clinical experts.

"Loving Lampposts" (2010):

The film delves into the controversies surrounding different autism treatments and highlights the various viewpoints on autism within the community.

"Life Animated" (2016):

This documentary is based on the book by Ron Suskind and tells the story of how Owen Suskind, who has autism, uses Disney animated films to communicate and connect with the world.

"The Reason I Jump" (2020):

Based on the best-selling book by Naoki Higashida, this documentary offers a unique and immersive insight into the experiences of non-verbal individuals with autism.

Social media platforms, such as Twitter (renamed X) and YouTube, have also become valuable spaces for individuals with autism to share their experiences, connect with others, and raise awareness about their challenges but also their strengths and achievements. By providing a platform for individuals with autism to express themselves, social media platforms have allowed for a more diverse and authentic representation of the autism community.

Chapter X

Behaviour

"Knowledge is *not* a *guarantee* of *good political behaviour, but ignorance* is a *virtual guarantee* of *bad behaviour"* - Martha Nussbaum.

I've been struggling to write this chapter and section of the book for nearly two weeks now. It's not due to writer's block, as thoughts bombard me constantly and inconveniently, like when I'm in the bath or picking up my daughter from school and when I can't record them on my phone. This week has been particularly challenging because it's February half term, and both my children are off school. My neurotypical teenage daughter is absorbed in her own world, interacting only with her online friends while playing Xbox and rarely engaging with me or anyone else outside her circle, except when she needs something. On the other hand, my son Rory, seeks my attention, and asks questions about the world.

Understanding Rory's unique needs and providing him with quality time has become a priority for me. Today, as we lay on the trampoline together, he surprised me by making new connections with the world around him. When I pointed out two airplanes flying overhead, he recognized them as planes for holidays. Later, we spotted a black and white magpie on our roof, and Rory referred to it as a penguin, reminiscent of a character from a children's program we used to watch together. Witnessing Rory's ability to recall details and make connections amazes me, especially considering his developmental delay. These moments of connection and growth are priceless.

After spending some time outside, jumping on the trampoline and installing a new garden hammock, we finally headed inside for a snack, as the skyline was turning grey and there was a likelihood of rain. It was then that I intended to start writing about why autism is a little like the weather and at times unpredictable and often different from what we expected our lives to be as parents.

For centuries, humanity has invested significant time and resources into predicting future weather conditions with only moderate success. The brain, like the weather, is a complex system influenced by various social, neurological, and environmental factors. This complexity makes it challenging to predict outcomes or define definitive future development for individuals diagnosed with any neurological condition.

Though I'm sure we've all experienced unpredictable weather events, like a sudden summer thunderstorm, despite the forecast predicting a sunny day. I recall the infamous hurricane that hit the south of England in October 1987. Back then, weather forecasts were limited to national TV, radio, and newspapers. The weatherman Michael Fish, during a live broadcast, infamously dismissed the possibility of a hurricane just hours before it struck. The storm caused significant damage, but as an eight-year-old at the time, I was more excited of an extra day off school. While weather forecasting has improved with advanced technology and data collection, it is still challenging to predict long-term weather accurately. Similarly, our understanding of autism has improved over the years, but there is still much we don't fully comprehend.

As parents, we have likely witnessed our child's unpredictable meltdown and crisis, just like that sudden unpredicted storm. Sometimes, we can't immediately identify the triggers or understand why our child's emotional state rapidly changes. But as neurotypical individuals we often filter out unwanted or unnecessary stimuli or information from our environments. If you've ever lived next to a busy motor way or railway line, you'll know what I mean. Whereas some autistic individuals are more attuned to sensory stimuli. Our children may sense and react to things that seem insignificant or undetectable to you or I.

Like Sherlock Holmes, we must become detectives, observing our child's behaviour, the situational circumstances, and the immediate environment to uncover the probable triggers and make any necessary adaptations. A trigger could be a change in noise levels, lighting, or other sensory factors, and as sherlock once said *"When you have eliminated all which is impossible then whatever remains, however improbable, must be the truth"*. During these early years, it's a journey of trial and error. We must find strategies to help our child adapt to a neurotypical world while also gradually developing their ability to filter out unnecessary sensory sensations or learn to adapt and mitigate. Tinted glasses or ear defenders can provide temporary relief during overwhelming situations, but it's important not to become overly reliant on them. Predicting outcomes becomes easier with experience, but it's crucial to remember that predictions are still just calculated guesses based on past events. As circumstances change, we must be prepared for that occasional storm that catches us off guard and without a coat or umbrella.

One such impromptu storm happened a few years back. Rory was preparing for an award evening, and he had felt immense pride when his teacher, Karla, nominated him for an achiever's award at the local MENCAP ceremony. MENCAP, formerly known as The Royal Society for Mentally Handicapped Children and Adults, was the association's new name. However, the actual ceremony posed a challenge as it was in an unfamiliar location and at a time when Rory typically relaxed in his bedroom. To prepare Rory for the evening, Karla and I discussed using the PECS (Picture Exchange Communication System) to help him understand the sequence of events. Although Rory preferred direct communication at home, I explained the same sequence using PECS to him over the week leading up to the ceremony.

The plan was for Rory to come home, have dinner, take a bath, skip bedtime, put on party clothes, drive to the party, meet his favourite teachers, and go home if he didn't want to stay. Rory not only understood this plan but also added his own requests. He wanted to take photos with his favourite people, carry his little yellow camera, bring his tablet for the journey, and carry his Minnie Mouse bag of toys and books.

The car drive went smoothly overall, despite a small hiccup when we initially went to the wrong location due to misplacing the invitation and instead relying on a Google search result. Once we reached the correct venue with ten minutes to spare, Rory got out of the car and headed towards the building with his camera in hand. However, he hesitated upon seeing the crowded foyer. This was expected, so we assured him that we would wait outside until the crowd went in. Our plan was to gradually help him reach the entrance of the foyer.

I had hoped that seeing Karla come round the side of the building, who was one of his favourite teachers, would encourage Rory to enter the building more willingly and quickly. However, that wasn't the case. As soon as Rory saw Karla, he began experiencing a crisis and meltdown. He dropped to the floor, threw his camera across the road, and kicked off his shoes as a means of distraction. Thankfully, we managed to intercept the shoes before they were lost. Despite our attempts to console and pacify Rory, he was determined not to go any further. Concerned for his safety and that of others passing by, I reluctantly decided to lift him onto my shoulder and carry him into the foyer, away from the busy road traffic. Using a fireman's carry/lift technique provided stability and prevented Rory from hurting me while also ensuring his safety.

Once inside the foyer, I gently placed Rory on the ground and reassured him repeatedly. However, he was beyond consolation at this point. He started kicking, pulling hair, hitting, slapping, and particularly scratching anyone near him. It became evident to all of us in the room that continuing with the evening wouldn't be fair to anyone, though especially Rory. We made one final request for him to put his shoes back on so we could return to the car and go home. Although it was challenging, we managed to get his shoes back on. Throughout the ordeal, I had to resort to a hold technique that I had previously introduced to Rory during tickle times. It was a last resort move to pacify him and prevent him from hurting himself and others. While holding him, I reinforced the concept that we express anger and unhappiness through hugs instead of hitting. The school also had a similar concept called a "Squeeze," which helped Rory release tension and anxiety.

Once Rory had his shoes back on, I informed him that it was time to get up and walk back to the car to go home. He complied, although he lashed out a few times during the process. He held our hands as we walked back to the car, with his older sister unfortunately getting hit before she could get inside. To prevent further incidents, I let her inside the car first, ensuring her safety. Once everyone was safely inside the car, I took a moment to catch my breath and assess the situation.

Rory was still upset and agitated in the backseat, displaying signs of distress and frustration. I understood that he had reached his breaking point, and it was important to give him the space and time he needed to calm down. I turned on some soothing music and spoke in a calm and reassuring tone to help create a more peaceful environment.

During the car ride home, I periodically glanced at Rory through the rear-view mirror, checking on his emotional state and making sure he was safe. I continued to offer verbal reassurance, letting him know that it was okay to feel upset and that we were there to support him. Once, we arrived home, I helped Rory out of the car and guided him to his bedroom, his familiar and safe space. I encouraged him to engage in his preferred calming activities, such as playing with his toys or listening to his favourite music. I stayed close by, ready to provide comfort and assistance if needed.

Over time, Rory began to relax and gradually regain his composure. I sat beside him, allowing him to take the lead in deciding when he was ready to talk or interact. I respected his need for space and ensured that he felt secure and understood. When Rory was ready, we discussed what had happened and acknowledged his feelings. I assured him that his emotions were valid and that it was okay to express them, but we also talked about alternative ways to handle his frustration that would be more constructive and safer for everyone.

In the days following the incident, I worked closely with Karla and Rory's school support team to develop strategies and techniques that would hopefully help prevent such overwhelming situations in the future. We focused on identifying and addressing the triggers that led to Rory's crisis and meltdown, as well as implementing proactive measures to support his emotional regulation.

Additionally, we scheduled a follow-up meeting with Rory's behaviour therapist to further assess the situation and determine any adjustments needed in his therapy plan. It was important for us to collaborate and share information to provide Rory with the best possible support and intervention.

As Rory's primary caregiver, I remained committed to understanding and advocating for his needs. I recognized that each situation was a learning opportunity, and it was crucial to adapt and refine our approach to ensure Rory's well-being and success.

Supporting individuals with unique challenges like Rory requires patience, empathy, and a willingness to continuously learn and grow. By working together as a team and tailoring our strategies to Rory's specific needs, we could help him navigate and thrive in various environments, gradually increasing his comfort and confidence over time.

Understanding Crisis / Meltdowns:

Many autistic children experience crisis, sometimes referred to as meltdowns, so it's essential to distinguish between your child's crisis and a temper tantrum. This basic guide is aimed at trying to help you anticipate, identify the causes of, and minimize the frequency of crisis behaviours in those you parent or care for.

What Is Crisis?

A crisis is an intense reaction to an overwhelming situation. It occurs when someone becomes entirely engulfed by their current circumstances, temporarily losing control of their behaviour. This loss of control can manifest verbally (shouting, screaming, crying), physically (kicking, lashing out, biting, throwing objects, hair pulling), or all of the aforementioned.

It's crucial to understand that a crisis is not a display of bad or naughty behaviour. When our child is utterly overwhelmed, and their condition makes it challenging to express themselves differently, a crisis is a natural discomfort or survival behaviour and akin to the fight or flight response.

A crisis is just one-way autistic individuals may express feeling overwhelmed. They might also withdraw from challenging situations or avoid them altogether.

What to Do During a Crisis:

If your child is experiencing a crisis or not responding, it's essential not to judge them. Providing support can make a significant difference to both your child and their other caregivers, should you be witnessing a crisis in public of someone else's child.

Give them time to recover from sensory or information overload.

Calmly inquire if they're okay, understanding that they may need more time to respond. Create a quiet, safe space, minimizing sensory input by reducing noise and bright lights. Encourage others to give space and avoid staring.

Anticipating a Crisis:

Many autistic individuals exhibit signs of distress before a crisis, often referred to as the "rumble stage." Signs may include anxiety-related behaviours like pacing, repetitive questioning, rocking, or becoming unusually still. During this stage, there's an opportunity to prevent a crisis. Strategies include distraction, diversion, offering calming tools like fiddle toys or soothing music, removing potential triggers, and staying calm.

Identifying the Causes:

A crisis results from overwhelming experiences. If you care for someone who experiences regular crisis events, identify what overwhelms them by keeping a record or diary over time. Record the events leading up to, during, and after each crisis. Patterns may emerge, such as specific times, places, or triggers.

Minimizing Triggers:

Once you've identified potential triggers, consider how to minimise them. While every autistic person is unique, common triggers include sensory differences, changes in routine, anxiety, and communication difficulties.

Sensory Considerations:

Many autistic individuals have sensory sensitivities, which can vary from over-sensitivity to certain senses to under-sensitivity in others. Tailor your approach based on their sensitivities. For example, if someone is sensitive to touch and sound, loud noises in crowded places like a shopping complex, supermarket or airport is likely to trigger a crisis. Consider using noise-cancelling headphones and timing your activities to avoid crowds.

Change in Routine:

Our children often thrive on predictable routines, so disruptions can be distressing. If a change is necessary, provide visual support explaining the alteration, offer reassurance about the rest of the routine, and include calming activities to ease the transition if possible.

Managing Anxiety:

The unpredictable world can cause anxiety in many individuals on the spectrum, potentially leading to a crisis. Try and develop strategies to manage anxiety, like creating a calming playlist, incorporating relaxation time into their routine, or using self-management support systems like the 'Brain in Hand app'. Having favourite toys as a distraction etc.

Communication Difficulties:

Your, child may struggle to express their needs, which can lead to overwhelming feelings or frustration. Support them in understanding and communicating their emotions before they become overwhelmed. Visual aids, social stories, communication systems, and modifying verbal communication may all be helpful.

By understanding crisis and their triggers, you can provide valuable support and create a more accommodating environment for autistic individuals in your life.

Chapter XI

Communication

"The most important thing in communication is to hear what is not said"- Peter Drucker.

Autistic individuals may exhibit various communication methods that may differ from typical verbal communication. Nonverbal communication plays a significant role for some individuals, utilizing gestures, facial expressions, body language, and eye contact (or lack thereof) to express their needs, emotions, and preferences. Echolalia, the repetition of words, phrases, or sentences heard previously, can serve as a communication method or a way to practice language skills for autistic individuals.

Another method is the Picture Exchange Communication System (PECS), where nonverbal individuals use pictures or symbols to communicate and make requests by selecting a relevant picture or symbol and giving it to their communication partner.

Augmentative and Alternative Communication (AAC) devices are also used, ranging from simple picture boards to high-tech electronic devices. AAC devices enable individuals with limited or no verbal communication abilities to express themselves through pre-programmed or text-to-speech messages. Sign language is another communication method employed by some autistic individuals, providing a visual and gestural way to convey thoughts, feelings, and ideas. Visual supports, such as schedules, social stories, and visual timetables, help individuals with autism understand and navigate their daily routines, providing structure, predictability, and clarity.

Specialized communication apps, designed specifically for individuals with autism, offer visual supports, picture-based communication, or text-to-speech features to facilitate communication and enhance social interaction. Sensory communication involves using objects, textures, or sensory experiences to convey needs, preferences, or discomfort. Additionally, social scripts in the form of pre-written or pre-recorded scripts assist individuals with autism in navigating social interactions, understanding social cues, and participating more comfortably in social situations.

Recognizing that communication methods could vary among autistic individuals, and what works for one person may not be effective for another. It is crucial to support and respect individual communication preferences, finding the methods that best suit their needs and abilities. Only the other night when I was sitting in the bathroom, I could hear two distinct sounds. The first is the unusual sound of my son crying, which doesn't fit with our usual routine. It's not caused by the common reasons like cutting his nails or hair tonight. I'll need to investigate as soon as I leave the bathroom. The second sound is that of my teenage daughter playing an online game, which is expected and in line with our normal household activities. It makes me contemplate the impact of social media and online gaming on communication skills. While they facilitate connections and networking, they also diminish our overall communication abilities. Some research suggests that 93% of daily communication is nonverbal, conveying messages through factors like facial expressions, gestures, and tone of voice.

The exact percentage may vary due to individual and situational factors, but the key takeaway is that nonverbal behaviour plays a crucial role in communication regardless of neurotypes. This is especially important to remember when dealing with individuals who are non-verbal or have difficulty speaking in conventional ways. Using precise terminology and descriptive words is often essential, as autistic individuals could interpret language literally. Misunderstandings can arise when phrases like "raining cats and dogs" are taken at face value. I recall a situation when at a party where an autistic woman took the phrase "help yourself to whatever food you want" literally and ended up taking all of one particular dish, unaware that it was meant to be shared. As parents, we need to be mindful of our choice of words and be explicit to avoid confusion.

In my own experience, I recently faced a challenge while explaining the concept of death to my son after losing my grandmother, his great-grandmother. I realized that my use of the word "dead" might have created a misunderstanding. Rory, like many autistic individuals, has become adept at using tablets or iPads for learning. When the device runs out of power, I often say it's "dead" and needs charging. As I explained death to Rory, I could imagine him visualising a scenario where we could simply plug his grandmother into a wall socket to bring her back to life. It made me realize the importance of choosing words carefully and finding relatable examples when discussing complex topics like death.

Returning to the present moment in Rory's room, it's evident from his body language and expression that he's unwell. However, he struggles to articulate his discomfort or specify its location. He can understand my questions but cannot provide a structured verbal response. We resort to a point-and-click adventure to identify the source of his pain, with limited success. Rory's inability to communicate precisely makes it challenging to address his needs directly, unlike neurotypical children who can express their discomfort verbally. We rely on visual cues and gestures, hoping to narrow down the possibilities of his ailment, such as toothache, sore throat, headache, cold, or earache.

Autistic individuals can often rely on non-verbal behaviour or alternative forms of communication when they cannot express themselves verbally. This can manifest as challenging behaviours that may seem abstract to us neurotypicals but serve as a means of communication. Rory, in the past, exhibited biting, hitting, scratching, and other undesired behaviours to express his reluctance or discomfort. Understanding and interpreting these forms of communication required us to step outside our familiar ways of verbal interaction and be more attentive to his non-verbal cues.

As morning arrives, I find myself sitting at the dining table, listening to Rory's cheerful singing. It brings a smile to my face, knowing that he is happy and content again. I often marvelled at his ability to recite lyrics perfectly while struggling with structured verbal sentences. A friend with a stutter once explained that singing bypasses the mental calculations and buffering required that a two-way conversation often involves.

There have been some wonderful, published books authored by autistic individuals that can explain their challenges firsthand and in a way, I can only empathise with due to not being autistic, but their accounts really should be recommended reading for any parent or caregiver that wishes to understand their child's communication challenges more.

"The Reason I Jump" stands as a remarkable literary achievement authored by Naoki Higashida, a profoundly talented writer from Japan who happens to be autistic. Despite facing substantial challenges in verbal communication, Higashida astoundingly captures his thoughts, emotions, and unique perspective on autism through his writing. Within the pages of his extraordinary book, Higashida offers profound insights into the inner world of autism, providing readers with a rare glimpse into the sensory experiences, social struggles, and intense emotions that individuals with autism often navigate.

Carly Fleischmann, a nonverbal autistic woman, harnessed the power of a keyboard to express her thoughts and feelings, offering invaluable insights into her experiences with autism through facilitated communication. Her remarkable work and writings have been recognized and featured in numerous publications and media outlets, serving as a beacon of understanding and inspiration.

Ido Kedar, another nonverbal autistic individual, has found his voice using a letter board and an iPad communication app. Through his written messages, Ido advocates for individuals who share similar experiences, empowering others and sharing his profound understanding of autism through books and public speaking engagements.

Tito Mukhopadhyay, a nonverbal autistic poet and author, defies the limitations of verbal communication through his powerful writings. Despite his nonverbal nature, Tito has authored several books that provide a unique perspective on autism, offering profound insights into his inner world. His writings have garnered critical acclaim, recognized for their immense impact on advancing the understanding of autism.

Sue Rubin, a nonverbal autistic woman, communicates using a keyboard and an augmentative and alternative communication (AAC) device. Through her articles, interviews, and personal accounts, Sue tirelessly raises awareness about nonverbal autism, contributing to the understanding and acceptance of individuals with limited verbal communication abilities.

DJ Savarese, a nonverbal autistic poet, writer, and advocate, utilizes a keyboard to communicate and share his powerful voice with the nonverbal autistic community. His writings, ranging from poetry to essays and articles, have been published in various literary magazines and anthologies, amplifying the voices of those who communicate through alternative means.

These exceptional individuals, each using their chosen modes of nonverbal communication, exemplify the profound impact of alternative methods of expression. Through their remarkable work, they have significantly contributed to the increased understanding, acceptance, and awareness of nonverbal autism, leaving an indelible mark on the autism community and society.

To provide support for nonverbal autistic children in the UK, it is essential to take a comprehensive approach that addresses your child's individual needs that promotes overall development and well-being. Early intervention services, such as speech and language therapy or occupational therapy, can be instrumental in providing tailored support to enhance communication skills, social interaction, and daily living skills.

Exploring Augmentative and Alternative Communication (AAC) options is crucial for empowering nonverbal autistic children to express themselves. Utilizing AAC systems like PECS (Picture Exchange Communication System), communication apps, or speech-generating devices can facilitate their ability to communicate, make choices, and engage in social interactions.

Visual supports, such as visual schedules, social stories, and visual cues, are valuable tools for enhancing understanding and providing structure. They assist nonverbal autistic children in navigating daily routines, comprehending expectations, and promoting communication.

Addressing sensory sensitivities is important, as sensory experiences can impact communication. Creating a sensory-friendly environment by managing triggers and providing sensory tools like weighted blankets, fidget toys, or sensory breaks supports self-regulation and comfort. Collaborating with the child's educational team to develop an Individualized Education Plan (IEP) that includes communication goals, strategies, and accommodations is essential. Additionally, supporting the development of social skills through structured training programs enables nonverbal autistic children to practice social interactions, turn-taking, joint attention, and understanding nonverbal cues.

It's critical that parents and caregivers seek out training and resources to enhance their understanding of autism and effective strategies for supporting nonverbal communication. Engaging in parent support groups and workshops provides opportunities to learn from others and share experiences. Finally, it is crucial to recognize and celebrate all forms of communication, valuing the child's unique communication style. Encouraging and validating their attempts to communicate creates a supportive and inclusive environment.

Always remembering that each autistic child is unique, and strategies should be tailored to their specific strengths, challenges, and preferences. Collaborating closely with professionals, educators, and therapists will provide invaluable guidance and support throughout the journey.

Chapter XII

Sleep

"When sleep is abundant, minds flourish. When it is deficient, they don't."
- Why We Sleep by Matthew Walker

Sleep challenges are common among autistic individuals, affecting not only the child but the entire family due to sleep deprivation. During the early years of Rory's life, he predominately slept in the same room as us. This was partly due to our limited living space, as we only had a two-bedroom home, and his older sister occupied the other room. Understandably, his sister's louder and more unpredictable bedroom routines may have made Rory hesitant to share a room with her. Additionally, during this time, Rory was pre-verbal, and his preferred mode of communication was through physical behaviours like hitting, kicking, biting, and hair pulling when he was upset. One subject that comes up with a lot of newly diagnosed children's parents is that of sleep.

Sleep difficulties can be prevalent among autistic children and can be caused by various factors. Sensory issues, such as sensitivity to noise, light, and touch, can disrupt their ability to fall and stay asleep. Additionally, anxiety, melatonin imbalance, certain medications, and medical conditions like gastroesophageal reflux disease (GERD) and sleep apnoea can contribute to sleep problems.

To assist autistic children in achieving a restful night's sleep, parents can implement effective strategies. Establishing a consistent bedtime routine, creating a peaceful sleep environment, addressing sensory issues through calming techniques or sensory tools, and considering melatonin supplements (under medical guidance) are proven strategies. Addressing medical concerns, ensuring a comfortable sleeping surface, promoting regular exercise, utilizing visual supports, managing anxiety, monitoring medication use, addressing behavioural issues, and exploring behavioural therapy options like CBT-I can also be beneficial.

By taking a proactive approach to improve sleep, parents can positively impact their child's behaviour, emotional well-being, and cognitive functioning, allowing them to thrive during the day and support their overall development.

I remember a significant sleep milestone occurring when Rory was twelve months old during our first camping trip. For the first time, he slept through the entire night for a full ten hours. Prior to that, he would wake up every four to five hours, wanting to get up, have a drink from his bottle, or engage with his surroundings. At the time, being relatively new to parenting and unaware of Rory's differences, I attributed his improved sleep on that camping trip to the fresh air and the outdoor environment. However, looking back, I realize that the change in routines and environment likely caused distress and confusion for Rory. The emotional turmoil and meltdowns he experienced on that first day exhausted him enough to sleep through the night. However, the tent and cool night air, along with the lack of electricity and electrical devices may also have attributed to a more suitable sleeping environment for him.

Hindsight has taught me the importance of learning from past experiences and problem-solving. Over the years, Rory's nighttime routines have become more consistent. He typically falls asleep early, usually between 7pm to 9pm, depending on the season and daylight hours. Once Rory is satisfied, he will lie down, fall asleep, and not wake up until morning. However, Rory's concept of morning was much earlier than ours, starting between 4 and 5 am, which felt like the middle of the night to us, but he's now learnt to amuse himself with a tablet until we collect him from his room to start his daytime routine. Regardless of whether it's a weekday, weekend, holiday, or special occasion, Rory always maintains the same sleep pattern.

Those with autism like any neurotype, might constantly have a lot on their mind. So, they may find it difficult to relax and let go, to be able to fall asleep, as thoughts and recollections from the day often occupy their minds at night. This often leads to two issues: difficulty falling asleep due to inability to relax and waking up in the middle of the night with anxiety. On the other hand, Rory has had little sleep problems related to his autism, perhaps as we identified the importance of this part of our lives was impacted more than others during those early days of pre and post diagnosis, and where perhaps the most work went into the importance of regulating a routine sleep pattern for Rory.

I remember reading the book "Why We Sleep" by Matthew Walker as a captivating and enlightening read of the science behind sleep and its vital importance to our overall well-being. Walker, a renowned sleep scientist, delves into the fascinating world of sleep, unravelling its profound impact on our physical and mental health. With a perfect blend of scientific research, personal anecdotes, and relatable storytelling, Walker takes you on a compelling journey through the various aspects of sleep, including its functions, dreams, and the consequences of sleep deprivation.

His book for me was packed with eye-opening revelations about the detrimental effects of insufficient sleep on our cognitive abilities, emotional resilience, and physical health, emphasizing the critical role sleep plays in our lives. "Why We Sleep" not only educates readers about the importance of prioritizing sleep but also offers practical tips and strategies for improving sleep quality. Overall, the book is a must-read for any parent interested in enhancing their or their child's well-being and understanding the profound impact that sleep has on our lives.

For a number of years Rory has followed his nighttime routine without trouble, once in his room, he's still very much not ready for sleep, but understands it's a time for relaxation and where the usual household sounds and movements are instead shut out from his space of safety and security that is his own bedroom. While in here and to satisfy his sensory needs, he would jump on his bed for hours, causing the ceiling to shake and dogs to bark. In the end we needed his bed to be reinforced and anti-vibration mats meant for washing machines to be placed under the bed's feet, not to mention the amount of mattresses we got through until settling on a rather costly all memory foam one.

If you get to the point of seeking assistance from your average GP, they will often prescribe Melatonin, However, it is not a miracle cure on its own and requires a consistent sleep routine to be effective. Melatonin is a hormone naturally produced by the body to regulate sleep and supplementing it can help establish a more consistent and restful sleep routine. For many autistic children, Melatonin supplementation has proven to be effective in reducing the time it takes to fall asleep, preventing nighttime awakenings, and improving overall sleep quality. By promoting a more regular sleep pattern, Melatonin may alleviate sleep-related challenges for autistic children and provide much-needed relief to both the child and their family. However, it is important to note that the use of Melatonin should always be done under the guidance and supervision of a healthcare professional and not purchased from the internet and the dosages guessed.

Joining an autism parenting group on social media and attending physical meetups around four years ago exposed me to the common topic of sleep and its challenges for both children and caregivers. Sleep is influenced by numerous factors, including timing, duration, and quality, and it plays a crucial role in our overall well-being. My most important advice is that everyone, including children, needs a good seven to eight hours of sleep every night to function optimally.

This can be a challenge for both children and parents at the beginning of their autism journey. Unfortunately, unlike other activities, the body cannot fully recover lost sleep, so it's essential to prioritise consistent and sufficient sleep.

To start to achieve a better night sleep for both you and your child, establishing a structured nighttime routine is key. Start by giving a warning about an hour before bed and engaging in the usual activities, such as brushing teeth and preparing a bottle or drink. If electronic devices are used in the bedroom, gradually reduce their usage over time, especially for devices emitting blue light, which can disrupt the onset of sleep. Ideally, create a dark and light-free environment in the bedroom, as darkness promotes the production of melatonin, the neurochemical that regulates our sleep-wake cycle.

For some of our children they may have difficulty understanding the need for sleep, so using visual supports like social stories or flow charts may help explain the process and provide reassurance. Some children like Rory may find the transition from sleeping in their parent's room to their own room challenging. This can be related to difficulty with change and a need for reassurance, with consistent reassurance and a creative approach to meet your child's needs may be necessary to address waking problems.

Keeping a sleep diary can be helpful in identifying patterns and factors that influence your child's sleep. It can also assist in tracking the effectiveness of sleep-related strategies and provide valuable information when seeking support from professionals.

As a parent, it's crucial to prioritize your own sleep as well. While it may be suggested to sleep when your child sleeps, this may not always be feasible. Creating a safe environment in your child's room will allow you to relax, knowing they cannot harm themselves while you sleep. Exploring community care and respite services and seeking support from professionals or your child's SEN school may also provide assistance when dealing with long-term sleep challenges.

Remember, sleep is essential for both you and your child's well-being. By implementing strategies and seeking support, you can gradually improve sleep patterns and promote better sleep for the entire family.

Chapter XIII

Food

"Let thy food be thy medicine and medicine be thy food".

- Hippocrates (400 BC)

Food presents challenges not only for the senses of texture, taste, and smell, but combined with the routines and rigidities of our child's needs it can be even more perplexing at times. Difficulties may arise as a matter of routine where trying new foods causes anxiety due to uncertainty. Many children have preferences such as not wanting different items to touch on their plate or eating items in a specific order. Some may stick to a particular colour of food, while others like Rory's breakfast choice may prefer Marmite or strong spicy flavours. The choice of eating utensils may also greatly impact their willingness to eat, with children demanding specific plates, cups or seating arrangements.

Generalization can also be problematic as like Rory, children may learn to eat certain foods only in specific places and struggle to apply that to other locations. Rory at home has a limited diet and is very specific about the foods he eats. Spaghetti Bolognese at school may be acceptable, but not at home. He has specific tastes and prefers bland foods with a particular texture. This makes it challenging when he goes visiting or when we are out and about, although we still have some options and manage to navigate through.

Selective eating refers to the unwillingness or inability to consume a wide range of foods, also known as "food neophobia" or "picky eating." Many individuals with autism have a limited diet and may restrict themselves to a small number of foods. Trying new foods or accepting alternative brands can be met with resistance. This can lead to nutritional deficiencies, weight fluctuations, and other health issues.

The subject of food and the process of selecting and consuming it may not seem challenging at first, but for those who haven't experienced raising an autistic child, it can become more complicated.

When choosing a new dish, you or I might typically rely on sight, smell, and asking about the ingredients. We use our sense of sight to identify the form of the food, whether it's solid or liquid. Then, we taste it to determine its flavour, whether it's bitter, sweet, or savoury. We can also sense the texture, whether it's hard or soft, and adjust our chewing accordingly. Apart from the initial selection, we go through these steps mostly subconsciously and without much thought. However, imagine the scenario I'm about to describe, disregarding cost and price as factors.

Picture yourself in a foreign country, such as Italy, dining out for dinner. You receive a menu with options like pizza, spaghetti and meatballs, or the local delicacy called "Pajata," which sounds interesting. The locals around you have ordered plenty of it, and as the saying goes, "When in Rome." However, you begin to wonder if it will be as tasty as it looks, considering you're not familiar with the exact translation of the menu's ingredients, primarily in Italian. So, you might decide to play it safe and choose spaghetti and meatballs.

Many neurotypical individuals would opt for a familiar dish like pizza or pasta, which we've had countless times back home in the UK. It's a safe option because we know what it looks like, and although the taste may vary slightly, it's familiar enough to enjoy. We tend to stick with this tried and tested approach, as most of us dislike change, which often brings a sense of risk. Since food is an important part of life, why take the risk of trying something different? Moreover, returning a dish because it's not to our liking can lead to embarrassment, social awkwardness, and anxiety when asking the waiter for a replacement.

The analogy above is perhaps not so different from the perspective of an individual with autism, particularly considering their heightened sensory input for sound, light, smell, taste, and textures. Taking risks with food can lead to anxiety, something that affects everyone but is especially prevalent in those on the spectrum. This anxiety for our children may also extend to familiar dishes prepared differently or in a different location. From various classes, talks, and literature, I've learned that food and its consumption can be challenging for some children on the spectrum. I've heard stories of children, including my own, who only eat one type of food. For example, I knew a boy who would eat any food as long as it was red in colour. Another boy, similar to a scene from the movie "The Imitation Game," would eat different foods but never if two vegetables were touching each other. My youngest stepchild, Apollo, is a more academically functioning autistic individual, and he follows a specific eating pattern where he systematically consumes his food in a particular order of preference. I've observed on many occasions that he always eats fries or chips first, followed by the burger, which he saves for last. I also have an autistic friend who's also diagnosed with attention deficit hyperactivity disorder (ADHD). He'll eats a variety of dishes, but they must all be drenched in a generous amount of burger sauce, which I should imagine makes everything taste practically the same.

There was a time when my own Rory would only eat solid, dry foods. Even mashed potatoes, with their butter and milk additions, were too close to a liquid form for him. For Rory to have managed baked beans back then was certainly out of the question, and it would almost certainly have ended up on the floor and then in the dog's stomach. Rory apparently now has a very varied diet at school. He'll eat fruits, vegetables, chicken korma, burgers, pizza, roast dinners, different desserts, and the list goes on. At home, however,

Rory refuses to eat anything besides homemade chicken nuggets and sausages with either gravy or tomato sauce for lunch and dinner. For breakfast, it's always Marmite on toast. Savoury food is always served on a Minnie Mouse plate, and sweet and snack food always on a Mickey Mouse plate. Cutlery—well, cutlery is negotiable, as Rory will often opt to use his fingers over a knife, fork, or spoon.

Due to his restrictive diet at home, and in order to try and get some vegetables and therefore vitamins in him, Jen and I will often resort to hiding blended vegetables into a thick gravy sauce or using liquid vitamin and mineral drops in his water or lemonade. But not too much of anything to give away our secret and alert him. As otherwise he'll watch you prepare the food or beverages to make sure you do it to his exact liking with none of your skulduggery involved. This method of sneaking ingredients into his food also works well for medicine dosages. So, if you are going to use this idea, be aware to transition changes gradually. Little and often is the recommended serving for such changes.

We once tried to replicate all the above school dishes at home, even going so far as to ask about the suppliers or the recipes used by the school's cook. We managed to loan one of the plates and trays they use, but Rory still wouldn't eat what we prepared. So, we currently continue with hiding ingredients in his gravy and drinks, knowing that at least at school he has a more varied and balanced diet.

Though a couple of weeks ago, Rory's teacher, Donna, and I were speaking on the phone when I happened to mention that Rory had stated to me during our routine conversation about school that they had made "Beans on toast in class." Donna said that Rory had enjoyed making the popular British snack but had refused to eat it after preparation. She couldn't understand why, as she had seen him eat both toast and beans during lunch on many occasions. I told her we had the same issue at home with introducing foods we knew he ate at school. Then the realization seemed to hit both of us at the same time as Donna said, "I wonder if Rory eats food associated with a certain place." BANG! She'd just hit the nail on the head. This made perfect sense. I knew that in certain restaurants, Rory would often eat a roast dinner, yet when at home, he wouldn't. Just like the school meals I had tried to copy, I had previously presumed that I had prepared it in a different manner or with different ingredients, which is why he wouldn't eat the home-cooked version. I was looking at this all wrong and from just a food point of view. When it was actually the surroundings in which Rory consumes different foods. Rory eats different foods in different environments. He works by association. Burgers at McDonald's, roasts at a carvery, school meals in the school canteen, and his very selective set menu at home. The environment, in this case, plays just as pivotal a role in his choice of foods as the food itself.

This revelation of thinking differently and by association led me back to a scene from the Temple Grandin movie biopic, in which Temple is mocked in a French language lesson for suddenly shouting, "Why are there so many fish in France?" Later, her science teacher, Dr. Carlock, discovers that Temple associates school subjects or any subject visually and in pictures. So, he relays his findings to his colleagues, particularly to the French teacher, opening one of Temple's textbooks to show hand-drawn pictures of eels eating at a table with a sentence underneath stating, "eels ate." The actual French words were supposed to be "ils est," which means in English "they are." Temple was visualizing the French word "ils" as the actual aquatic animal, an eel. Carlock explains that language is difficult for Temple to grasp as it's obviously not as visual a subject as something like woodwork. This revelation leads the other teachers to adapt their subjects where possible to Temple's visual learning style, and voila, they see academic improvements in Temple.

The benefit of finding a local SEN parenting group was also highlighted in another fantastic book ironically named "Toast". This book has a chapter on associated food strategies and the challenges the British author Alice Boardman encountered while raising her two autistic sons, Tom, and Alex. Alice herself mentions that Alex had a habit of eating off the carpet. Unable to find a way around this, Alice serves Alex's meals on the carpet for him. One day at a parent's group, she overhears another mother in a similar situation to her own, where the woman's son ate off the carpet. But this mother had remedied this by using a carpet sample as a placemat at the dining table. What a simple and obvious solution to a challenge that most of us might simply overlook. Alice also makes a very good point that I feel like I should highlight here, and that's that sometimes it doesn't matter how much or how often you try something new; your child just might not be in the right place in time for them to tackle a new food or challenge. It's not until our children age that we, as their parents, might actually start to understand them a little more, and we're able to start seeing the signs when they are more receptive to new ideas. Only then might we try and seize the moment by working to encourage them to try something new. After all, even as a neurotypical individual, I have only just started to re-try food and beverages I previously disliked in my younger years, such as coffee, Branston pickle, and some spicy foods. When I was younger, I simply wasn't ready, either mentally or physically, as our sense of smell and tastes often change as we hit middle age, and our taste buds may decrease and shrink.

Gastrointestinal (GI) problems may also be prevalent among autistic individuals. These problems may include constipation, diarrhoea, and abdominal pain. The exact causes of GI issues are not fully understood, but disruptions in the gut-brain axis, and communication network between the gut and brain, may play a role and could significantly impact individuals' quality of life. Selective eating and food aversions can result in limited dietary choices, leading to malnutrition or weight-related problems that further impact GI problems and cause additional discomfort and may require medical intervention.

There are several interventions available to help address eating behaviours associated with autism. One common approach is food chaining, which involves gradually introducing new foods that resemble those already accepted by the individual. While sensory-based feeding therapy focuses on addressing sensory sensitivities through controlled exposure to different textures, smells, and tastes.

Additionally, dietary interventions like the gluten-free and casein-free (GFCF) diet may benefit some individuals with autism, although its effectiveness varies among individuals.

So, addressing eating behaviours of autistic children can present challenges. Particularly those with limited communication abilities that make it difficult to identify underlying causes. Interventions often require substantial time and resources, with any outside therapy often requiring multiple sessions or implementing dietary changes. Additionally, the lack of standardization and evidence-based research on interventions poses difficulties in determining the most effective approaches.

I've gained insights from both reading and experimenting with Rory that certain children might find it challenging to consume natural foods like fruits and vegetables due to the varying aspects of taste, smell, shape, and colour each piece presents. In contrast, processed foods such as chicken nuggets offer a sense of predictability, where each chocolate biscuit is identical to the next, creating a reassuring familiarity. Nevertheless, many of these processed foods fall into the category of ultra-processed foods and beverages (UPF), which is a complex issue in itself. Some studies have suggested a potential connection between UPF consumption and ADHD behaviours as well as mental health concerns.

The World Health Organization has cautioned that neglecting mental health conditions during adolescence can have enduring repercussions into adulthood. Recent research indicates that around 1 in 7 (14%) adolescents encounter mental health issues, with conditions like depression, anxiety, and behavioural disorders ranking among the primary contributors to illness and disability. Thus, it's imperative to identify additional factors that interact with mental health problems, with a particular focus on devising preventative strategies for adolescents.

Diet quality plays a crucial role here, and a poor diet characterized by high consumption of UPF could be a modifiable risk factor for mental disorders. For a deeper understanding of UPF and its impacts, irrespective of neurotype, I suggest exploring "Ultra-Processed People: The Science Behind Food That Isn't Food" by Chris van Tulleken. Chris, a father, scientist, doctor, and esteemed BBC broadcaster, offers valuable insights on this subject.

Hopefully by understanding some of the challenges associated with food, you'll be able to hopefully consider the challenge of introducing new varieties of food. If you are new to the challenges of food and just starting your own journey with your child on the spectrum, my only advice will be to keep trying. Don't give up trying new strategies or revisiting old ones. Eventually, like everything, time is the main ingredient here, along with a pinch of persistence, a spoonful of patience, and seasoned with plenty of love.

Chapter XIV

Toileting

Life's a piece of shit, when you look at it, Life's a laugh and death's a joke, it's true.. – Michael Palin: Monty Pythons, Life of Brian.

The enlightenment of my previous conversation with Rory's teacher, Karla, about his association with food led me to envision another problematic area of our daily life together with Rory, which was toileting. Rory now has no problem using the toilet to urinate and defecate at school, it seems. But at home, he would only urinate during the day. Rory would categorically refuse to come out of nappies at night, always opting to defecate once or twice in his nappy during bedtime. We knew he didn't like the sensation of having a soiled nappy, as he would stand about in his room waiting to be changed. We also knew that during camping holidays, Rory would use a porta-potty or compact camping toilet at night. So, he was capable of using a toilet in the twilight hours but obviously wasn't doing so at home. Discovering that Rory is more likely to adapt via association to his given environment meant that the solution, for now, has been to use a camping toilet in his bedroom. Rory started to use the toilet within hours of its introduction without any protest or prompting, and now two weeks later, he continues to do so. For hygiene reasons, this isn't the most practical solution, especially with the warm summer months coming and the risk of smells escaping the toilet and into his room. Rory is very sensitive to smell and will often retch, dry heave, or vomit if the smell is too much for him. But like the introduction of blended foods in Rory's diet, slight adaptation with gentle change is likely the key for us moving forward with his nightly toileting or, in this case, a sideways movement towards the actual bathroom toilet.

For parents starting their own journey. The internet and social media can be a minefield of information, especially the subjects and strategies associated with food or even toileting. But for me personally, it's been better to find a local group of similar parents and chat about the challenges they too may or may not have encountered themselves. As I've stated previously, you need to allow time to start connecting all the dots. And there is possibly no better way to do this than to speak to others in a similar situation or those who at least have a good understanding of an autistic child in general, such as an educator of those with special needs.

Toilet training can be a challenging process for parents of autistic children, as there can be various difficulties related to sensory sensitivities, communication, and physical issues. It's important to understand and address these challenges to support your child effectively.

One common difficulty is knowing when to use the toilet and how to communicate their need. Our children may have trouble understanding verbal instructions or expressing their toileting needs clearly, so creating visual supports like picture schedules or visual charts might help them grasp the process better and reduce anxiety.

Sensory sensitivities can also play a role, making the bathroom environment overwhelming for some children. Considering factors like lighting, noise levels, and smells can create a more calming atmosphere.

Addressing sensory preferences for toileting materials, such as toilet paper or soap, is crucial to ensure your child feels comfortable during the process.

Establishing a consistent toileting routine and using positive reinforcement can help motivate your child. Praising and offering rewards when they successfully use the toilet can reinforce positive behaviours.

Functional communication methods like using gestures or signs can empower your child to express their toileting needs effectively. Breaking down the toileting process into smaller, manageable tasks can make it less overwhelming for your child and help build their confidence.

Toilet training aids, like adaptive toilet seats or step stools, can promote independence and comfort during toileting time.

Modelling and peer support can be helpful, showing your child appropriate toileting behaviours. So, perhaps lead by example and show them the process yourself if it's a process you haven't yet explored. Practice sitting on the toilet as part of their daily routine without immediate expectations to wee or poo. Avoid repetitive toileting strategies that may become unhelpful or boring for the child. Encouraging your child to participate in the toileting process, like pulling down pants or washing hands, fosters independence.

Monitoring fluid intake is essential, especially if your child struggles to recognise bodily signals indicating the need to use the bathroom.

Gradually transitioning your child towards using the toilet, even if they start with their nappy on, can aid them in adapting to this new behaviour. We applied this strategy when moving Rory's portable camping toilet closer to the bathroom. Initially, we placed it in the hallway, then on the landing outside the bathroom, and finally, we positioned it inside the bathroom next to the actual toilet before eventually eliminating it entirely.

Above all, patience and understanding are crucial. Some children may have difficulty comprehending the social expectations of toileting, requiring adaptation and guidance in different settings as Rory still presently does, as we can attest during our recent trip back from Cornwall, we made a stop at a Moto services to take a break and use the restroom. However, as soon as Rory stepped out of the vehicle, he attempted to pull down his shorts and pants to urinate in the open grass and pavement. This situation posed a potential problem, with several people, including families with young children, in close proximity. While this behaviour might be acceptable for a toddler, it was not suitable for a twelve-year-old boy who was already showing physical signs of puberty. I immediately intervened and stopped him. I understand his confusion, considering that during our holiday, we often took walks in natural settings like forests, beaches, and rivers, where we would simply find a discreet spot behind a tree or boulder to relieve ourselves when necessary. Now, it seemed like I was changing the rules, saying 'No' just because others were around. Thankfully, Rory didn't strongly protest when we explained that we needed to use the indoor toilets due to the presence of people. He followed Jennifer to the restrooms without much resistance. However, the look of confusion on his face highlighted the challenges our children face in social settings and the need to adapt our behaviours accordingly. Sometimes, individuals with autism may not comprehend the potential consequences of seemingly harmless actions, which can quickly escalate into serious and hostile situations, especially when we, as parents, are not there to address and explain their actions. I can't help but imagine the ramifications if he were older, say 16 or 18, and accidentally exposed himself innocently in the presence of a young girl aged ten or less. Therefore, we've employed various strategies over the years, but even then, like in this recent incident, new challenges may arise.

Teaching your child proper toilet use can be a challenging task, regardless of whether they are on the autism spectrum or not. However, the process of establishing a toilet routine may take longer and come with its unique challenges like it did for Rory and us to find something that worked.

This guide aims to provide you with practical steps to help make toilet training a success –

When to Begin:

Choose a time when you have fewer commitments and feel relatively stress-free to start the toilet training process. Some indicators that it's a good time to begin include:

- When your child starts showing awareness of the need to go to the toilet.
- If you notice changes in their behaviour, such as distraction or fidgeting when they are wet or soiled.
- When they communicate their need for a diaper change.
- If your child is aware of their bathroom activities (starting/finishing urination or bowel movements).
- When your child displays an interest in using or has used the toilet without prompting.
- If your child can hold their urine or bowel movements for one or two hours at a time (improved bladder/bowel control).

Developing a Toileting Routine:

Keep in mind that achieving independent toileting is the ultimate goal, and it may take several months with numerous small successes along the way. Aside from the physical aspects of toilet training, consider social factors. Many autistic children may not have the social motivation to imitate adults or peers in using the toilet, especially after using nappies or diapers for an extended period like Rory had. Always remembering that each child is unique, and different teaching techniques may be needed.

Our children appreciate routine. So, use that to leverage their desire for predictability to establish a successful toilet training routine.

Here are some steps:

- Change your child's diaper in the bathroom to associate toileting activities with this location.
- Avoid using a potty to prevent a challenging transition from potty to toilet.
- Ensure everyone involved in your child's care begins toilet training simultaneously and follows the agreed-upon approach. Send necessary equipment to school, such as a toilet seat reducer.
- Observe your child's bathroom habits over a few days to identify patterns that can increase the likelihood of successful toilet use.
- Continue taking your child to the toilet at set times based on your observations. If they have an accident, get them to the toilet quickly, and praise them for what goes in the toilet.
- Utilize a visual sequence next to the toilet to help your child understand the expected steps, which can be in the form of photographs, pictures, or written words.
- Ensure that instructions and images are clear to prevent misunderstandings.
- Follow a consistent sequence of behaviours each time to create anticipation and make your child more receptive.
- Focus on addressing one behaviour at a time, as changing multiple behaviours at once can be challenging.
- Determine how to praise your child for successfully following the toileting routine, considering their preferences for social praise or tangible rewards.

Dressing and Undressing:

Dress your child in comfortable, easy-to-manage clothing, such as elastic waistbands and shorter dresses or skirts.

Encourage underwear use by selecting pairs featuring their favourite characters.

- Use the "backward chaining" technique to teach new skills, breaking them down into smaller steps and allowing your child to complete the final step independently.
- Hand Washing
- Maintain a consistent hand-washing routine with clear steps.
- Stand behind your child and physically guide them, gradually withdrawing assistance.
- Minimize verbal prompts and provide a visual sequence as a reminder.
- Consider teaching your child to use the cold tap to prevent burns in unfamiliar settings.

Boys, Sit or Stand:

Decide whether to teach a boy to sit or stand to urinate based on his ability to distinguish between urination and bowel movements, coordination, and the availability of someone to imitate. In our case, we followed the school's approach, so we had Rory sit for both. It wasn't until much later, perhaps two or three years after he had mastered seated toileting, that Rory suddenly discovered he had an appendage that could more easily aim streams of urine while we were out camping or on a hike, away from public amenities.

- To teach aiming, place a target (e.g., a piece of cereal) in the toilet for them to focus on. Fun toilet target stickers are also available online. Whatever you decide to use in the toilet, try to make sure it's something biodegradable. While colourful

Lego pieces may float and make fantastic targets, using them poses a risk of both toilet clogs and environmental harm, as they are not biodegradable and could potentially enter the watercourse and harm wildlife much later during wastewater treatment. Instead, if colour motivates your child, consider using fruit or vegetable skins (e.g., red apple, green apple, banana, or orange peels).

Bowel Control:

- Bowel control typically follows on from bladder control. Some children find bowel movements frightening, so use visual aids or books to explain the digestion process.
- Address the sensory aspect of a full nappy-diaper by finding alternative ways to provide comfort.
- Transition from using a nappy-diaper with a hole cut in the bottom to eventually going without it to help your child feel secure and relaxed on the toilet.

Habit Training:

- Habit training involves taking your child to the toilet at specific times throughout the day to create a routine.
- Observe your child's natural patterns to determine the best times for toilet trips.
- Ensure your child is relaxed enough to urinate or have a bowel movement while on the toilet.
- Use toys or objects to keep your child engaged and relaxed during toilet time.
- Teach your child a strategy to avoid accidents, such as counting to ten before getting up.

- Consider using vibrating watches or home electronic devices to give an audible cue to help your child manage their toileting routine independently.

Creating a Comfortable Environment:

- Make the bathroom a calm and relaxing space for your child to encourage independence and success in the toileting routine.
- Eliminate distractions unrelated to toileting.
- Ensure comfort with foot supports, side rails, and a smaller toilet seat.
- Adjust everything in the bathroom to your child's level, including soap and towels.
- Address sensory needs by considering factors like scent, noise, water temperature, and lighting.
- Ensure your child can sit comfortably on the toilet with their feet flat on a secure object.

Night-Time Toilet Training:

- Start night-time toilet training once your child is mostly dry during the day.
- Establish a consistent bedtime routine, including limiting fluid intake before bed.
- Take your child to the toilet before bedtime and potentially once during the night.
- Use protective bedding products.

Schools and Early Years Settings:

- Remember that admission to school should not be denied based on continence issues, as this may constitute disability discrimination. Whatever strategies are already in place within an academic or home setting should remain consistent across all settings, so habits and routines remain the same regardless of the change of location.

Additional Tips:

- Offer a drink 10 to 15 minutes before toilet time to encourage urination.
- Decide whether your child should learn to close the door as part of their toileting routine or in specific situations.
- Avoid using childlike terms for toileting to ease language transition.
- Address any fears your child may have, such as flushing the toilet, by adjusting the routine or using calming methods.
- In the car, provide a protector for the car seat and limit drinks before long journeys.
- Be aware that some children may wait for a diaper to release their urine or bowel movement.
- Explore absorbent pants and swimwear options for older children.
- Once your child is toilet trained at home, teach them to use public toilets by following a consistent routine and using familiar visual aids.

Chapter XV

Education

"Education is the most powerful weapon you can utilize to transform the world." – Nelson Mandela

Growing apprehension surrounds the provision of education for children with special needs, as recent data reveals an unprecedented surge in complaints upheld by England's government ombudsman this year. An analysis of these decisions exposes a distressing situation: some children with special educational needs and disabilities (SEND) have languished without a school placement for over a year. This surge in complaints is unfolding against the backdrop of the SEND system grappling with increasing demand and years of inadequate funding. Across England, local councils are grappling with substantial deficits in their SEND budgets due to protracted delays in issuing Education, Health, and Care Plans (EHCPs). These EHCPs delineate the educational support that children with the most pressing needs should receive, but sadly, these stipulations are frequently left unmet.

The number of complaints upheld by the government ombudsman regarding special needs education has soared by over 60% since the previous year. From the outset of 2023 to mid-July, the Local Government and Social Care Ombudsman (LGO) either partially or fully upheld 380 complaints, a stark increase compared to the 234 upheld complaints during the same period the year prior and 167 until mid-July in 2021. This surge persists despite constraints in capacity, prompting the ombudsman to adopt a more discerning approach to the cases it investigates.

A spokesperson for the SEND Action campaign group remarked, "The substantial uptick in complaints upheld by the ombudsman is compelling evidence that the SEND crisis is spiralling beyond control. The penalties imposed for failing to meet legal obligations pale in comparison to the cost of delivering services, and unfortunately, some local authorities are exploiting this situation, resulting in a dearth of accountability that detrimentally affects young disabled children, and their families. There has been a conspicuous dearth of government action, including under the SEND and alternative provision plan, to augment accountability and ensure that local authorities align with their legal responsibilities."

Many of these grievances are linked to delays stemming from a shortage of educational psychologists (EPs), whose assessments are integral when councils formulate EHCPs.

Research published by the Department for Education (DfE) earlier this summer revealed that 88% of councils are grappling with EP recruitment challenges, with a third encountering hurdles in retaining them.

The current AEP General Secretary Cath Lowther stated, "Despite the indispensable services and support provided by EPs, local authorities are failing to invest in the profession, leading to widespread recruitment and retention difficulties. The resulting surge in EP workloads means that children and young people are enduring excessively long waits for EP consultations or, even more regrettably, are denied these consultations altogether."

The findings recently heightened the financial redress that councils are obligated to provide, increasingly urging them to enhance their services to prevent other parents from encountering similar predicaments. Local governments and the social care ombudsman, commented, "Complaints related to SEND, especially those concerning Education, Health, and Care Plans, remain a primary focus of our work, characterized by one of the highest rates of upheld complaints. Complaints concerning education and children's services represent some of our most prominent cases, and over the past year, we have issued more reports on these areas than any other."

Every child deserves access to an education that fosters a joyful childhood, promotes positive outcomes, and prepares them for adulthood and potential employment. Recent improvement plans delineate how they intend to reform the support system for children with SEND, while fostering consistent high standards nationwide and ensuring that parents do not have to wrestle for access to support. While there has been a substantial increase to investment in the high-needs budget, with an additional £440 million earmarked for 2024/25, bringing total funding to £10.5 billion, representing a rise of over 60% since 2019/20.

However, regardless of our child's needs finding the right school for our children can be challenging whatever their abilities, this challenge can become somewhat harder if they are diagnosed before or around school starting age. Because until they start to develop, you may not fully understand their challenges or potential, and making the wrong school choice, as we did, can make finding a suitable placement difficult due to the limited availability of special educational needs schools, which are often oversubscribed with long waiting lists.

Despite my initial disregard for Rory's challenges or differences, luck was on our side. The challenges he faced at the nursery led to early referral services and a diagnosis before he was due to transition into infant school. Originally, he was supposed to follow his sister to a school that suited her needs, and we immediately put Rory's name down to attend as well. The headmaster, a direct and formal man, genuinely cared about the children's academic and social well-being. He took time to attend meetings between the nursery, relevant local authorities, and made his assessment that even with additional funding for a learning support assistant (LSA), the school wouldn't meet Rory's needs, which, though shocking at the time, prevented him from being placed in the wrong setting, for which I'm forever grateful.

Rory's late August birthday meant that he not only had additional needs but would also be among the youngest in his academic year, potentially putting him at a greater disadvantage. So, with input from various agencies, we decided to keep Rory at the nursery a little longer while his diagnosis was underway, and a 'Statement' *(now more commonly replaced by an educational, health, and care needs and provision or EHCP)* could be prepared to address his academic needs. Fortunately, the diagnosis and statement were relatively quick, giving us an idea of his educational requirements, which meant we needed to explore different special needs schools in the area.

During our first school visit, I was taken aback by the severity of physical and mental needs some children exhibited. I remember stating, "Rory's not that bad; I don't think he'll be coming here. He's not going to be as affected as some of these children." Moreover, the headmistress intimidated me with her blunt manner, and I doubted Rory would respond well to her or the staff. Looking back, I realize how naive I was, and was later to discover that this was actually the perfect setting for Rory to not only be content within an academic environment, but to have also prospered there and he continues to do so in the present.

At that time we considered various schools, such as profound and multiple learning disability (PMLD), severe learning difficulties (SLD), and moderate learning difficulties (MLD). However, we were unaware that different schools offered varying levels of education and support based on the child's learning difficulties. To us, they were all SEN schools and therefor the same, and we made our selection based on what we witnessed when visiting, and the promises made during what were essentially sales pitches. My understanding at the time was limited to Rory's speech difficulties, and I believed he could eventually handle GCSE-level subjects and proceed to college and university.

Hence, we chose a MLD school in Thundersley, Essex, but unfortunately, things didn't start well. Rory wasn't settling in, and his outbursts and behaviour worsened despite our hopes that he would adjust to the new environment and routines. By the end of the summer term, the school questioned whether this was the right setting for Rory, but they still decided to keep him in the same class for the new academic year due to his half-year absence. The next year, his outbursts and echolalia persisted, leading him to lash out at his peers and causing other parents to complain about their children's well-being and belongings. The school's solution was to isolate Rory from his classmates, why still failing to address some of the underlying issues associated with his behaviours. One of the factors that influenced challenging behaviour was the school assembly held in the school hall, a situation they were aware posed a challenge for him because of the noisy surroundings when many students gathered in one place simultaneously. I tried to convey to them the difficulties of such environments and shared some strategies I had utilized, as well as the gradual progress we had achieved in addressing this specific challenge. However, it became evident that my input was not given due consideration, possibly perceived as unwarranted meddling from just another parent who believed they comprehended the situation better. The class teacher persisted in employing a methodology reminiscent of ABA (Applied Behaviour Analysis) to address the challenging behaviours exhibited by autistic children. ABA relies heavily on structured repetition, with a primary focus on applying reinforcement to encourage desirable behaviours and deter undesirable ones. This reinforcement can encompass both positive and negative strategies, and similarly, punishment can take both positive and negative forms. In essence, ABA therapy in autism strives to make a child fit into a more 'normal' or neurotypical mold, rather than acknowledging that certain behaviours are intrinsic to an autistic individual. Consequently, ABA therapy limits an autistic child's autonomy over their environment and fails to fully embrace sensory aids like headphones, sunglasses, fidget toys, weighted blankets, and more. Even when these supports are allowed, they are frequently utilized as incentives with time constraints rather than serving as genuinely beneficial sensory tools. Consequently, existing in an environment that employs planned neglect (ignoring a child during distress or crisis-meltdown), declines to accommodate their sensory sensitivities, and instead rewards them for concealing their sensory discomfort can potentially result in trauma and long-term harm. In essence, ABA attempts to compel autistic individuals to endure or disregard their challenges, essentially masking their differences in a world oriented towards the neurotypical paradigm of conformity and acceptance.

Ultimately, after a few more months Rory faced permanent exclusion from the school due to what is commonly cited as "persistent disruptive behaviour." This outcome was quite unexpected for me, especially considering it was a SEN school, though I now think that the headmaster's interpretation of SEN actually meant "Selective Needs School" when it came to Rory's challenges.

Subsequently, Rory's exclusion drastically reduced his educational support, leaving him with only two hours of one-on-one tutoring each week. This was a stark contrast to the previous 30 hours of education he had received, along with additional emergency funding for extra one-on-one classroom support.

I found myself perplexed by the decision-making process of both the school and local authorities. It remains a source of confusion, especially when you consider that every school in the UK receives a per-student funding allocation, which can be further augmented for children with additional needs. Despite my less-than-stellar math skills, I couldn't reconcile the financial resources the school received, including the emergency funding, with the budget allocated for Rory's one-on-one tutoring sessions outside of the school premises. These sessions certainly weren't taking up money on hiring a space as a dedicated classroom or learning facility, as the tutor often had to work within limited spaces provided by a library or health centre, or wherever was available on Rory's tutoring day.

This presented its own set of challenges since, as any parent of an autistic child knows, changes in location and environment frequently trigger anxiety in our child. This meant that constant changes in the learning environment often set Rory and his tutor up for a challenging day. This form of lacklustre alternative education was also only provisioned for 20 sessions.

Realizing that we had most definitely chosen the wrong school for Rory, we explored other options, including SLD (Severe Learning Difficulty) and PMLD (Profound and Multiple Learning Difficulty) schools. Although there were only three such schools in our area, one was grossly oversubscribed, and another was the same school we had initially dismissed for not being suitable because I didn't initially believe Rory was as profoundly affected by his autism as much as I cared to believe. However, this school was undergoing rebuilding to better accommodate students' needs and offer more spaces, and it would be this school that he still resides at currently. But it meant more than twelve months of exclusion or sufficient provisions made toward his lack of education.

So, after spending more than a year outside of SEN education, Rory finally secured a placement at the very same school we had dismissed when first selecting suitability two years earlier, which had now been rebuilt to include modern amenities and a larger capacity of learners. The school's philosophy towards learners and learning was markedly different from that of his previous school, and they handled inappropriate behaviours with compassion during moments of crisis. Rory has thrived in this school and remains content and settled there. He affectionately refers to his friends and teachers as "Rory's People," which always brings a smile to my face, as if he were a Roman senator addressing his people in a colosseum.

The various acronyms, abbreviations, and initialisms used in diagnosis by medical clinicians, the local authority, and academic settings can be quite daunting, especially for parents who are new to a diagnosis. It wont be uncommon to see report of messages reminiscent of the following: *"Child (X's) (ASD) and their need for an (ECHP) and (EP) in addition, (child X) may require some assistance from (NELFT) before enrolling the child in a (PMLD) (SEN) school"*

To help ease this confusion, here are some of the more common definitions of Special Educational Needs and Disabilities (SEND) that you may encounter, along with some of the more common comorbidity (additional condition/s) associated with autism that you may encounter in an EHCP or EP referral.

Comorbidity:

Comorbidity refers to the concurrent presence of one or multiple additional diseases or disorders alongside a primary disease or disorder. A comorbid condition represents a secondary diagnosis with core symptoms that differ from those of the primary disorder. Comorbidity is notably more prevalent among autistic individuals when compared to the general population. To illustrate, individuals with autism are 1.6 times more inclined to experience conditions such as eczema or skin allergies, 1.8 times more prone to develop asthma and food allergies, 2.1 times more susceptible to frequent ear infections, 2.2 times more likely to suffer from severe headaches, 3.5 times more at risk of experiencing diarrhoea or colitis, and 7 times more likely to report gastrointestinal (GI) issues.

(Source- Al-Beltagi, Autism medical comorbidities 2021)

Dyslexia:

Dyslexia primarily affects accurate and fluent word reading and spelling. It involves difficulties in phonological awareness, verbal memory, and verbal processing speed. Dyslexia varies in severity and may co-occur with other language, motor, and organizational difficulties.

Dyscalculia:

Developmental Dyscalculia is a specific learning difficulty characterized by impairments in learning basic arithmetic facts, processing numerical magnitude, and performing accurate calculations. These challenges must be significantly below expectations for an individual's age and not caused by poor education, daily activities, or intellectual impairment.

Dyspraxia:

Pupils with dyspraxia experience difficulties in controlling or co-ordinating movement, which can affect activities like writing, typing, and speech.

Education, Health, and Care Plan (EHCP):

The process of obtaining an (EHCP) for a child with special educational needs, including autism, can be lengthy and complex. In the past, it could take several months to complete the assessment process, gather necessary evidence, and draft the EHCP.

Echolalia:

Echolalia is the involuntary repetition of another person's speech and is particularly common in young children as part of language development. However, if it persists past the age of three, it may indicate speech or developmental delays. Echolalia can be immediate (repeating right away) or delayed (repeating after some time) and can be categorised as communicative (with a purpose) or semi-communicative (without a clear purpose), and is frequently observed in autistic individuals, with up to 75% of children displaying the behaviour. Additionally, echolalia can be a feature of Tourette syndrome (TS), a neurological disorder characterised by motor and vocal tics.

Educational Psychologists (EPs):

Educational psychologists play a crucial role in helping children and young people reach their full potential by working in partnership with local authorities, families, and other professionals. They use their psychological training and knowledge of child development to assess learning difficulties and offer guidance to schools on how to support children's learning and development effectively. They stay updated on best practices, policies, and research related to child learning, influencing local policies and practices.

Educational psychology services may vary by region, with schools or groups of schools typically assigned an educational psychologist or team. A practice agreement outlines the services provided throughout the school year, ensuring it meets everyone's needs.

Children may come to the attention of educational psychologists through various means, such as early years assessments, teacher concerns, or parent requests. Assessments are ongoing and integrated into the learning and teaching process. Educational psychologists gather information from teachers, parents, observations, and discussions with the child, if appropriate.

They support schools in considering the holistic needs of children, provide advice to school staff, offer training, and assist in communication between schools and parents. Educational psychologists also work with families of young children and help plan transitions for young people entering employment or further education.

While they offer recommendations regarding school placements, the final decision lies with the local authority. Parents have the right to request a specific school placement and can appeal if their request is denied.

Executive Functioning (EF's):

Executive functioning refers to a set of cognitive processes that are responsible for planning, organizing, initiating, completing, and adapting to tasks and situations. These functions help individuals manage their daily lives and achieve goals effectively. In the context of autism, executive functioning can be affected, and individuals with autism spectrum disorder (ASD) may experience challenges in these areas.

Speech, Language, and Communication Needs (SLCN):

Children and young people with speech, language, and communication needs (SLCN) face challenges in effectively communicating with others. Their difficulties may lie in expressing themselves, understanding spoken language, or comprehending social communication rules. Each child's SLCN profile is unique and may evolve over time, affecting different aspects of speech, language, or social communication.

Individual Education Plans (IEPs):

IEPs are written by the school usually when a child is on Stage 2,3,4 and 5 of the Sen Code of Practice. An IEP is a detailed plan that sets out targets and strategies to help your child learn. An IEP will usually contain three or four individual, short-term targets for your child to focus on.

North East London Foundation Trust (NELFT):

NELFT is an NHS foundation trust which provide an Emotional Wellbeing Mental Health Service for children and young people across the whole of Essex. We are the provider of all age eating disorder services and child and adolescent mental health services.

Moderate Learning Difficulties (MLD):

Pupils with MLD have attainments significantly below expected levels across various subjects despite interventions. They may struggle with basic literacy, numeracy, understanding concepts, and exhibit delayed speech and language development, low self-esteem, and social skill underdevelopment.

Profound and Multiple Learning Difficulty (PMLD):

Pupils with PMLD have severe and complex learning needs, often combined with physical disabilities or sensory impairments. They require extensive adult support for both learning and personal care. The curriculum is broken down into small steps to accommodate their needs, and communication may be through gestures, eye pointing, or symbols.

Severe Learning Difficulty (SLD):

Pupils with SLD have substantial cognitive impairments affecting their ability to participate in the curriculum without support. They may also experience challenges in mobility, co-ordination, communication, and self-help skills. Pupils with SLD require support in all curriculum areas, and some may communicate through signs, symbols, or simple language.

Social, Emotional, and Mental Health Difficulties (SEMH):

Children and young people may exhibit various social and emotional difficulties, including withdrawal, disruptive behaviour, or challenging actions. These behaviours can indicate underlying mental health issues like anxiety, depression, self-harming, substance misuse, eating disorders, or unexplained physical symptoms. Some individuals may have specific disorders like attention deficit disorder, attention deficit hyperactivity disorder, or attachment disorder.

Specific Learning Difficulties (SpLD):

 SpLD encompasses a range of learning differences across pupils. They may have specific difficulties in reading, writing, spelling, or manipulating numbers, and these challenges may be more pronounced than in other areas of learning. Short-term memory, organizational skills, and co-ordination can also be affected.

The only guidance I can offer is based on my own experiences and the challenges faced by Rory. However, with the benefit of hindsight, I would have opted for a school catering to Severe Learning Disabilities (SLD) or Profound and Multiple Learning Disabilities (PMLD) from the beginning. If it turned out that Rory was not suitable for that environment and was a more capable learner, than in my experience, it would have been easier to transition towards schools focused on Moderate Learning Disabilities (MLD) or mainstream education and not the other way around. This approach is preferable because specialized SEN schools are relatively scarce across the UK and often oversubscribed.

So, my advice to parents who may have doubts about their child's academic abilities is to consider the worst-case scenario where their child might struggle with learning and social communication. It is essential to be honest with oneself and avoid overestimating or assuming your child's potential academic abilities as I once did. Making the wrong decision can lead to heartache and significant challenges for the entire family unit, not to mention impacting the child's education and overall well-being.

Chapter XVI

Health & Hygiene Tips

"The greatest wealth is health." – Virgil

Pain and Discomfort

A recent study provides insights into how adults diagnosed with autism perceive and respond to painful stimuli.

Tseela Hoffman and her research team examined pain perception in a group of 104 adults, of which 52 had been diagnosed with ASD. These autistic individuals, ranged in age from 18 to 55, were carefully matched with neurotypical controls based on age and sex, and both groups displayed similar performance on a cognitive assessment.

The researchers discovered that autistic participants were more inclined to use psychiatric medications. Furthermore, they self-reported higher levels of anxiety and heightened sensitivity to pain and other sensory inputs.

During sensory tests, both participants with autism and the control group exhibited similar thermal and pain detection thresholds, suggesting normal functioning of the peripheral nervous system in autism. However, when exposed to various stimuli surpassing their pain threshold, autistic individuals consistently rated their pain as more intense compared to the control group, indicating hypersensitivity to pain. The study also revealed that those individuals could effectively inhibit brief pain stimuli but struggled to do so with long-lasting pain stimuli.

In summary, the researchers proposed that autistic individuals exhibited a "pro-nociceptive" pain modulation profile, implying that their brains appear to be more active in amplifying the experience of pain while being less effective at inhibiting prolonged pain. This profile may increase the risk of these individuals developing chronic pain. The researchers also highlight that their findings align with the theory suggesting that autistic individuals may have an imbalance between neural excitation and inhibition.

Conclusively, the researchers argue that their evidence, which demonstrates heightened sensitivity to pain, challenges the common misconception that autistic individuals experience less pain. This misconception could lead to delayed diagnosis and inadequate treatment, resulting in increased suffering and potentially exacerbating autistic symptoms such as sleep disturbances, restlessness, and aggressive behaviours.

Dental Care

Rory's avoidance of dental care and his reluctance to sit in the dentist's chair are concerning issues. Despite having been to the dentist before, we've only managed to get him to open his mouth briefly for a visual inspection. His teeth brushing routine is also far from adequate, lasting no more than ten to fifteen seconds.

Approximately six months ago, we noticed significant facial swelling on one side of Rory's face, which leads us to suspect it might have been caused by an abscess. Surprisingly, Rory has never mentioned any discomfort or pain associated with his mouth, but it is evident that he needs some form of examination and possible corrective treatment if there's an underlying issue.

To address Rory's dental needs, we've sought a referral to the community dental service, which caters to individuals with specific needs who cannot access care from a general dental practitioner. Unfortunately, the waiting time for an appointment is quite long, around twelve months or even more.

When Rory finally receives treatment from the community dental service, they will likely administer anaesthesia to ensure he's unconscious during any necessary dental work. Due to the possibility of extended gaps between visits, they might choose to remove his tooth rather than attempt complex procedures like root canals that require multiple visits.

As Rory's caregivers, it is our responsibility to support him through this process. We need to communicate openly with him about the importance of dental health and address his fears and concerns. By offering gentle encouragement and seeking professional advice, we can gradually help him improve his oral hygiene habits.

Moreover, exploring behavioural techniques and considering mental health support can aid Rory in coping with his dental anxiety. We should lead by example, demonstrating good oral hygiene practices to show him that dental care is essential and nothing to fear.

Ultimately, we hope that by working together with Rory and the community dental service, we can ensure he receives the necessary dental care and prevent any further complications. Our aim is not only to address immediate concerns but also to empower Rory to take charge of his oral health and well-being in the long term.

Finger & Toenail Trimming

Trimming Rory's fingernails has proven to be an even more challenging task than cutting his hair. I vividly remember an incident a couple of years ago when we attempted to get his feet measured at a Clarks shoe store for the new school term. Despite the store's efforts to make adaptations by providing seating outside and having a salesperson assist with the measurements, the experience overwhelmed Rory, and Jen still carries the literal scars of that challenge, with what looks like an Asian Kanji symbol etched into her forearm.

Besides ourselves, Rory's long fingernails had caused concern for his educators and peers at school. When he's upset, he tends to scratch and gouge those around him, sometimes leaving marks on people if his nails are not kept short. This prompted us to realize that proper nail care was essential for everyone's safety and well-being.

Initially, we used to pin him down on the ground and carefully trim his nails with the help of a second person. However, as he has grown older, so has his strength, making it increasingly difficult to continue with this method. The whole experience was miserable for all of us, and we knew we had to find a better approach.

Thankfully, the school has made steady progress in helping Rory tolerate having his fingernails trimmed with nail clippers. This year has marked a significant improvement in his ability to communicate when and how he needs his nails trimmed. As a result, the process has become less distressing for everyone involved.

It has taken a total of three years for the school to introduce the nail clippers gradually. They began by letting the clippers touch only the tip of his finger during class group activities, where all children participated. Over several months, they progressed to cutting multiple nails, and this continued under different teachers and teams. Thanks to their patient approach, Rory is now comfortable with having his fingernails cut, but his toenails remain too sensitive for a complete trimming session. Instead, if a particular toenail is broken and causing him discomfort, he will ask us to trim it.

The acknowledgment and success of this challenge are truly owed to the school and their fantastic team for their ongoing dedication to Rory's progress.

Here are some tips recommended on how to best handle this task, but they are pretty much the same repeated approaches to all the challenges I'll cover in this chapter:

Prepare the environment:

Choose a quiet and comfortable space where your child feels safe. Minimize distractions and ensure good lighting.

Explain the process:

Before starting, communicate with your child about what you're going to do. Use social stories, simple language and visual aids if needed, so they can understand what to expect.

Use appropriate tools:

Select nail clippers that are safe, easy to handle, and have rounded edges to reduce the risk of accidental cuts.

Start with short sessions:

Initially, trim only one or two nails at a time to help your child get used to the sensation and process gradually.

Offer choices:

Allow your child to choose which hand you will start with or which nail to trim first. This sense of control can make the experience more empowering for them.

Provide sensory support:

Some children may benefit from sensory input before or during the process. You can offer them items like a stress ball or fidget toy to hold.

Distract with preferred activities:

Engage your child in an activity they enjoy while you trim their nails. This can help keep them focused on something positive and lessen any anxiety.

Consider alternative methods:

If using traditional clippers is too distressing, explore other options like electric nail files or emery boards. Choose the method that your child feels most comfortable with.

Praise and reward:

Offer positive reinforcement and praise for each successful nail trimming session. You can also provide small rewards to further encourage cooperation.

Be flexible:

If your child is not receptive during a particular session, try again later or on another day. It's essential to be patient and understanding of their needs.

Always remembering that every child is different, and what works for one may not work for another. It may take time to find the best approach for your child, just as it did for Rory but with patience, consistency, and a supportive attitude, you can help them become more comfortable with nail trimming over time.

Hair

In the earlier years, giving Rory a haircut was quite a challenging task. It involved me embracing him tightly to prevent any sudden movements or crying fits, as he would often experience a crisis and try to escape. Afterward, we would all be left exhausted from the ordeal. At that time, this was the only method that seemed to work for this bi-annual task. However, as time passed and strategies evolved, especially in the last couple of years, Rory has become more open to getting his hair cut. In fact, he now reminds us when his hair is getting long by stating, "My hair's long, it needs to be cut."

Undoubtedly, this experience is still difficult for him to endure, but he has learned to tolerate it. Like many other challenges we've faced together, it's been a journey of trial and error, with more errors than successes along the way. Presently, the most acceptable way of cutting his hair is in a location of his choosing, which has included the outdoor trampoline in the past. To help distract him during the process, he usually has a tablet or iPad to keep him engaged.

A couple of years back, a breakthrough came when Jen suggested using dog or pet hair clippers, as they are quieter than their human equivalents. However, we still encounter difficulties when cutting around his ears, an ultra-sensitive area for Rory. For this part, we have to resort to using scissors or conventional trimmers while he's asleep to achieve a tidy cut.

Cutting the hair of an autistic child can be a challenging task, as it involves sensory experiences and potential anxiety triggers. Again, with patience, understanding, and a thoughtful approach, you may be able to create a positive and comfortable haircutting experience for both your child and you.

Here are some tips to tackle cutting hair for an autistic child that others have also used:

Preparation is Key:

Before starting the haircut, take the time to prepare the child for the experience. Use social stories, visual schedules, or picture cards to explain the haircutting process step-by-step. Familiarize the child with the tools you'll be using, such as scissors or clippers, and let them handle these items beforehand if they feel comfortable.

Gradual Desensitization:

Before using the clippers on the child's hair, introduce the buzzing sound gradually. Turn on the clippers at a distance and gradually bring them closer to the child. This process can help desensitize them to the noise and vibration.

Use Noise-Cancelling Headphones:

These have never worked for Rory as his ears and the area around them are ultra-sensitive for him, but you could try and provide your child with noise-cancelling headphones or ear defenders to reduce the intensity of the buzzing sound. The headphones can create a calming environment and help the child feel more in control during the haircut.

Offer Sensory Distractions:

Introduce sensory distractions to divert the child's attention from the buzzing sensation. Providing fidget toys or stress balls can help them focus on something comforting while the haircut is underway.

Visual Supports:

Use visual supports like social stories or picture cards to prepare the child for the haircut. Illustrate the steps involved in the process, including the use of clippers. This visual aid can help the child anticipate what to expect and reduce anxiety.

Respect Their Limits:

Be prepared to modify your approach or try different techniques if the child becomes too distressed. It's crucial to prioritize the child's comfort and well-being above completing the haircut quickly.

Seek Professional Support:

If the child's sensitivity to buzzing sounds remains a significant challenge, consider seeking help from an occupational therapist or specialist experienced in working with autistic individuals. They can provide tailored strategies to support the child during haircuts.

Choose a Calm and Familiar Environment:

Select a quiet and familiar place for the haircut, preferably a location where the child feels at ease. Minimize distractions and noise that could overwhelm the child during the process.

Sensory Considerations:

Be mindful of the child's sensory sensitivities. Provide options for sensory tools, like fidget toys or weighted blankets, to help them self-regulate during the haircut. Experiment with different types of hairdressing capes or aprons to find one that feels comfortable for the child.

Communication and Breaks:

Maintain open communication with the child during the haircut. Use simple and clear language to explain what you're doing and check in with them frequently to ensure they feel comfortable. Allow the child to take breaks if needed to reduce anxiety.

Remember, that all our children are unique, so what worked for Rory may not work for your child. Be patient and flexible in your approach, and always prioritize the child's comfort and well-being, don't do as I did and manhandle and force the issue. Instead, celebrate even the smallest successes, and over time, the child's experience with haircuts may become more positive and manageable.

Hearing

Parents and caregivers of autistic children often encounter distinct challenges in identifying and addressing hearing difficulties, particularly due to communication and expression struggles that many autistic children experience. Recognizing hearing issues in such cases can be even more complex.

I realized that Rory's hearing had only been tested during his diagnostic phase. This experience was quite intriguing, considering how much hearing tests have evolved since my own school days when we simply used headphones and signalled when we heard sounds of different frequencies. Rory's hospital hearing test aimed to rule out deafness as one of his communication obstacles. However, getting him to the hospital and awaiting the test was quite stressful. Rory's distress and headbanging in response to the overwhelming and noisy hospital environment almost led us to call it off and return home. Luckily, just as we were about to give in, we were called into the testing room. The test involved Rory sitting in a room with puppets popping out of the wall or appearing from behind a screen, each accompanied by a sound. As the test progressed, the sounds were mixed with visually distracting toys. This innovative method allowed for observation of Rory's responses to familiar sounds associated with specific toys, prompting him to look in the direction of the expected toy, whether it appeared or not. This modern 'Visual Reinforcement Audiometry' (VRA) testing approach that combines visual cues and associated sounds is exceptionally beneficial for very young infants or children with social communication difficulties. It provides valuable insights into their hearing abilities and aids in understanding their responses in a more interactive and engaging manner.

By understanding the signs, available tests, and recommended strategies, I hope to equip parents and caregivers with valuable tools to support their child's hearing health effectively. Recognizing

155

Potential Hearing Difficulties: The first step in testing hearing difficulties in autistic children is to be vigilant for signs that may indicate a problem. Since communication may differ in autistic individuals, it is essential to look beyond conventional indicators like responding to their name or following instructions.

Some potential signs of hearing difficulties in autistic children include:

- Limited or delayed language development
- Difficulty understanding spoken language or responding appropriately to conversations.
- Heightened sensitivity to certain sounds or environments
- Lack of reaction to loud noises
- Repeatedly asking for information to be repeated or misunderstood instructions.

Consulting with Professionals:

If you suspect that your autistic child is experiencing hearing difficulties, seeking the guidance of healthcare professionals is crucial. An audiologist, speech-language pathologist, or an ear, nose, and throat (ENT) specialist with experience in working with autistic children can help you navigate this process. They will conduct a thorough evaluation to determine the extent of your child's hearing challenges.

Audiological Tests for Autistic Children:

Audiological tests are essential for assessing hearing abilities in autistic children. However, traditional tests like pure-tone audiometry may not be suitable due to the child's developmental differences. Instead, the following modified tests can be used:

Visual Reinforcement Audiometry (VRA):

This test uses engaging visual stimuli to encourage the child to respond to sounds, even at a young age.

Play Audiometry:

Utilizing play-based techniques, this test assesses the child's responses to sound stimuli during interactive games.

Conditioned Play Audiometry (CPA):

Similar to play audiometry, CPA involves linking specific actions with sound responses to evaluate hearing capabilities.

Communication and Accommodation:

Effective communication with autistic children during the testing process is vital. Utilize visual supports, such as pictures or gestures, to facilitate understanding. Patience and flexibility are key when dealing with their unique sensory needs and communication styles. Additionally, ensure that the testing environment is comfortable and accommodating, minimizing potential sensory distractions.

Testing hearing difficulties in autistic children requires a comprehensive approach that acknowledges their individuality and communication differences. By being vigilant for potential signs, seeking professional help, and utilizing modified audiometric tests, we can better understand and address hearing challenges in our children. Empowering parents and caregivers with knowledge and empathy is the first step towards ensuring that every child receives the best possible care for their hearing health and remembering that early identification and intervention play a critical role in supporting their overall development and well-being.

Medication

In this section, I'll cover both how we tackled administering medication to Rory. Secondly, I will discuss perhaps some of the common medications that you may encounter or learn about through sources such as parents of autistic children or individuals on the autism spectrum themselves.

Administering Medications:

Getting Rory to take any kind of medication when he was just a toddler proved to be an incredibly challenging task, akin to attempting to give a cat oral medication or a bath. It often required the efforts of two people, with one person wrapping Rory in a bath towel to prevent him from struggling and lashing out, while the other person attempted, usually unsuccessfully, to coax him into taking a spoon or syringe in his mouth. More often than not, the medication ended up anywhere on his face except in his mouth, and occasionally, it even landed on our faces as he spat it back out.

Fortunately, we quickly discovered an effective solution that we still use today for Rory's anti-anxiety medication, as well as for administering anti-histamines for insect bites and liquid pain relief. Now, we simply conceal the medication in his beverage or mix it with strongly flavoured paste or liquid food, such as his morning marmite on toast, flavoured water, yogurt, or even in his daily gravy served with homemade chicken nuggets. This method is particularly convenient when the medication is in liquid form. Otherwise, we crush it into a powder.

Another important consideration is the medication's concentration. It's crucial to ensure your child consumes the entire dose in one go, especially if it's mixed with a small amount of food or drink. For Rory, I typically offer a half-slice of marmite toast containing the medication, and once he's finished that, I provide the rest of his breakfast. If you plan to use this approach, always consult your pharmacist to ensure there are no interactions or adverse effects when combining the medication with the chosen food or beverage.

But that's it, that's our tactic for navigating Rory's aversion to medications. He's still none the wiser but gets what he needs when he needs it.

Sleep Disorder Medication – Melatonin:

Melatonin, a hormone originating from the pineal gland in the brain, governs the body's diurnal (day and night) circadian rhythms, orchestrating the sleep-wake cycle. The process begins with the retina's perception of light, which signals the suprachiasmatic nucleus (SCN) in the hypothalamus, the part of the brain behind circadian rhythms. In response to darkness, the SCN prompts the pineal gland to craft melatonin from tryptophan, commencing in the evening hours. Melatonin is then released into the bloodstream, reaching various regions of the brain, including the hypothalamus, where it activates receptors, promoting drowsiness and triggering the onset of the sleep cycle. Melatonin also exerts influence over core body temperature, contributing to the rejuvenation of restorative sleep. This natural orchestration ensures our sleep patterns harmonize with the day-night cycle, ushering us into slumber as evening descends and awakening as morning beckons.

Melatonin's history is noteworthy: Before 1995, it was readily available as a dietary supplement in health food stores. However, it underwent a reclassification as a medication, and in the UK, it can now only be obtained through a prescription. Nevertheless, individuals are legally permitted to import melatonin for personal use from countries where it remains unrestricted. Curiously, many US and Australian online vendors such as Amazon and eBay offer melatonin products to UK customers. Similar to my later explanation regarding the purchase of CBD edible and oil products in the UK, I would caution against seeking melatonin from online retailers. The primary reason being that some online remedies lack regulation, making it difficult to ascertain their true concentrations and dosages, if they are accurately labelled at all.

Before considering medical intervention or prescribed medications, the initial step for children should be to maintain consistent sleep routines synchronized with circadian rhythms. This is pivotal for several compelling reasons. The circadian rhythm, often referred to as the body's internal clock, governs the sleep-wake cycle and influences various physiological processes. In children, particularly infants and toddlers, adhering to regular sleep patterns will aid in establishing healthy sleep habits, promoting optimal brain development, and supporting overall physical and emotional well-being. Disruptions to these routines can result in sleep deprivation, which, in turn, may impact cognitive function, mood regulation, and even physical growth. By adhering to a consistent sleep schedule that respects natural circadian rhythms, parents and caregivers can provide a sturdy foundation for children to flourish, nurturing enhanced sleep quality, improved daytime functioning, and overall development.

Furthermore, both electronic devices and room temperature wield substantial influence over the quality and duration of sleep. Electronic devices emit blue light, which can suppress melatonin production, the hormone regulating sleep, thus disturbing the body's natural circadian rhythm, and hindering the ease of falling asleep. Additionally, engaging with stimulating content or checking emails on these devices before bedtime can elevate cognitive arousal and delay the onset of sleep, frequently leading to a reduction in overall sleep duration. On the other hand, room temperature assumes a pivotal role in shaping a comfortable sleep environment. The ideal room temperature for sleep generally falls between 15 to 19 degrees Celsius (60 to 67 degrees Fahrenheit). A room that is excessively warm or cold can cause discomfort and awakenings during the night, interfering with the body's natural temperature regulation, which entails a gradual decrease in core temperature as it prepares for sleep. Maintaining a cozy thermal setting is instrumental in supporting the body's natural sleep-wake cycle and fostering rejuvenating sleep.

Anti-Anxiety & Anti-Depressants Medications –

The discussion about the use of anti-anxiety medication was somewhat contentious between Phoebe and me during Rory's time with her amid our separation. Phoebe struggled to manage some of Rory's challenging behaviours both at home and outside, including daily routines and new or altered schedules. She had heard from other parents that ADHD medication might alleviate some of these behaviours she was witnessing, as she thought he might have that condition in addition to ASD. I reluctantly agreed to at least consider the idea, and we scheduled an appointment with the same paediatric consultant who had initially diagnosed Rory with autism.

I recall Phoebe being visibly upset as she explained to the consultant that she was struggling and believed that medication might help, just as it had helped other parents, she knew whose children also had autism, some with an additional diagnosis of ADHD. The paediatrician attentively took notes and waited for Phoebe to finish and regain her composure. Then, he turned to me and asked how Rory behaved when he stayed with me and Jennifer. It was strikingly different from what Phoebe was describing – almost as if we were talking about a completely different child. While Phoebe encountered significant challenges in her interactions with Rory, we occasionally encountered hesitancy or resistance, but not the full-blown crisis-meltdowns and physical altercations that she described when dealing with similar situations.

The paediatrician then inquired, "Do you think it's the environment?" I replied, "It's either the physical environment or the individuals within that environment." This seemed to strike a nerve with Phoebe, as if I were personally attacking her. "I'm not lying, Matt. You can ask the school," she retorted. Phoebe was correct; at that time, Rory had just started school and was facing difficulties there as well. The school reported similar challenges, although perhaps not as intense as what Phoebe was experiencing at home.

I wasn't questioning the validity of her reasoning for considering medication or Rory's challenging behaviours. I was simply pointing out that Jennifer and I weren't encountering the same behaviours as Phoebe or the school. I said, "Ask Rose (his sister) how he is with me; she'll tell you he's not as difficult as you're describing." This was another truthful statement, and Phoebe was well aware of it. However, by this point, she was exhausted from having to struggle with Rory for the simplest tasks, such as putting on shoes, only for them to end up tossed out of the car when the door or window was open. Many shoes, socks, toys, books, and electronic tablets had met their demise on road trips.

The only time I experienced some of the behaviours Phoebe described was when I needed to return Rory to her after he had stayed with me. Predictably, this was when we would witness full-blown crises-meltdowns, from the hallway to the front door, in the street, in the car, and throughout the journey to his mother's house. It was emotionally and physically exhausting, and I'm not a small person. So, if this was the same behaviour Phoebe was dealing with – and she is barely five feet tall – then I completely understood why she sought help in any form, whether it be therapy, medication, or some other unknown strategy.

The paediatrician turned to both of us and said, "I don't believe Rory has ADHD and I don't think he needs medication, and without further assessment and referral, I can't prescribe any." This was a significant setback for Phoebe, as it left her wondering where to turn next. As mentioned in earlier chapters about relationships and education, Rory's challenges became so frequent and overwhelming for both Phoebe and his school that he was eventually permanently excluded from his SEN school. This led to extended periods at home, where his challenging behaviour continued to escalate, prompting local government intervention. Eventually, the decision was made for me to take over his daily care, and he was eventually reintroduced to a more understanding SEN academic setting around 2017.

However, all our lives globally were upended again in early 2020 due to COVID-19. When Rory returned to school after the worst of the pandemic had passed in 2021, he struggled once more with the transition back into education. Although the challenges were not as severe as before, and we still did not witness them at home, the school noticed a pattern of anxiety, often linked to the absence of classmates or educators. Unlike his previous school and Phoebe, the new school identified a pattern and a trigger, allowing them to implement various techniques to manage Rory's anxiety when changes occurred unexpectedly in the classroom. Some techniques worked better than others. The school also noticed that Rory's anxiety often escalated into physical crises, typically between 1 and 3 pm after lunch. They tried several techniques with moderate success.

At this point, I was convinced that enough evidence had been gathered, and the behaviour patterns were predictable enough to warrant an assessment by an educational psychiatrist. Consequently,

Rory was prescribed an anti-anxiety and anti-depressant medication called Sertraline. Incidentally, this was the same medication I had been taking since my mental health deteriorated, leading to a breakdown in 2015. I remained steadfast in my belief that medication should always be a last resort for managing behaviour, including my own erratic choices during periods of depression and anxiety. Because of my history with the medication, I had already thoroughly researched Sertraline, including its effects and side-effects, so I was aware of how it might affect Rory, given that we shared some of the same physiological characteristics as father and son.

Like any medication, it took time to determine the correct dosage. As Rory matures and grows physically, he will require annual reviews to assess whether the medication remains effective. Since beginning Sertraline in 2021, Rory has shown improvement in handling changes within academic settings, particularly those related to his friends and other students, as well as the absences of teaching assistants and teachers due to illness or holidays. Previously, when someone was absent, Rory would become fixated on that absence and would be unable to focus on other tasks while his anxiety continued to escalate. Since starting the medication, Rory has been better equipped to cope with the absences of classmates and educators. While the anxiety is still present, it is more manageable for him and the school staff, allowing them to effectively mitigate his anxiety and worries with more success.

Some of the most common anti-anxiety medications prescribed for autistic children in the UK include:

Citalopram and Sertraline both are- Selective Serotonin Reuptake Inhibitors (SSRIs):

Benefits:

SSRIs are commonly prescribed for anxiety disorders in autistic children. They work by increasing the levels of serotonin, a neurotransmitter associated with mood regulation, in the brain. Benefits may include reduced anxiety, obsessive-compulsive behaviours, and repetitive thoughts.

Side Effects:

Common side effects can include nausea, upset stomach, sleep disturbances, and in some cases, increased agitation or irritability. In rare cases, SSRIs may be associated with an increased risk of suicidal thoughts or behaviours in children and adolescents.

Buspirone (Buspar):

Benefits:

Buspirone is a non-addictive anxiolytic medication used to treat generalized anxiety disorder. It can be beneficial for managing anxiety symptoms in autistic children.

Side Effects:

Side effects may include dizziness, headaches, nausea, and nervousness.

Atypical Antipsychotics (e.g., Risperidone):

Benefits:

Some atypical antipsychotic medications, like Risperidone, may be prescribed to manage severe anxiety, aggression, or irritability in autistic children. They can help reduce certain behavioural symptoms.

Side Effects:

Potential side effects include weight gain, increased risk of type 2 diabetes, and movement disorders.

Benzodiazepines (e.g., Diazepam, Lorazepam):

Benefits:

Benzodiazepines are fast-acting medications that can provide short-term relief from acute anxiety or panic attacks.

Side Effects:

They are generally not recommended for long-term use due to the risk of dependency and side effects like drowsiness, dizziness, and impaired coordination.

Beta-Blockers (e.g., Propranolol):

Benefits:

Beta-blockers may be prescribed to manage physical symptoms of anxiety, such as rapid heartbeat and trembling. They are less commonly used in children but can be considered in specific cases.

Side Effects:

Side effects may include fatigue, dizziness, and lowered blood pressure.

The decision to use medication should always involve a comprehensive discussion with a qualified healthcare professional, taking into consideration the child's unique needs and circumstances.

It's crucial to note that medication should only be considered after a thorough evaluation by a qualified healthcare professional. The benefits and side effects of medication can vary from child to child. In many cases, behavioural interventions, therapy, and environmental modifications are recommended as the first line of treatment for anxiety in autistic children. Medication is typically considered when these approaches prove insufficient or when anxiety symptoms are severe and significantly affect the child's daily life.

Families and caregivers should closely monitor any child on medication, and regular follow-ups with healthcare professionals are essential to assess the effectiveness and safety of a treatment.

Non-Prescription Anti-Anxiety / Sleep Aid Medication – CBD:

In 2018, the poignant media headlines featuring Billy Caldwell and Alfie Dingley shed light on the irrational and inhumane challenges faced by parents of children grappling with severe epilepsy in the UK. This distressing situation stemmed from outdated policies surrounding cannabis-based medicines. Both sets of parents asserted that cannabis oil played a crucial role in managing their children's seizures, yet they encountered official prohibitions and even had their oil confiscated. Only recently have government officials started engaging in discussions regarding the imperative need to reevaluate these policies.

During this period of heightened media scrutiny, Jen pondered the potential use of cannabidiol oil, more commonly referred to as CBD oil, to help alleviate some of Rory's anxiety when confronting new challenges, such as navigating unfamiliar environments or meeting new people. I harboured reservations regarding the authenticity and potency of numerous over the counter and online suppliers operating in the market.

So, for those less informed, what exactly are cannabis oils? Cannabis oil is derived from the Cannabis sativa plant, renowned for its medicinal properties for over 3,000 years. It found mention in the ancient Egyptian Ebers papyrus around 1550 BC and likely served as a remedy in China even earlier. Some strains of this plant contain significant levels of tetrahydrocannabinol (THC), the psychoactive compound responsible for the "high" associated with smoking or consuming cannabis leaves or resin. Another major constituent of the plant is cannabidiol or CBD, which is devoid of psychoactive effects. Both THC and CBD interact with the body's natural cannabinoid receptors, influencing various processes like memory, pain perception, and appetite. Additionally, the cannabis plant contains over 100 other cannabinoids, albeit in lower concentrations. Whether cannabis oil can induce a high would depend on its THC content. Some varieties of the Cannabis sativa plant, termed hemp, contain negligible levels of THC. Extracts from these plants consist predominantly of CBD and do not produce a high. This is crucial, especially when considering the application of such remedies to children.

In addition to epilepsy, cannabis-based medications are available for various other conditions. Nabilone, a synthetic form of THC, has been in use since the 1980s to combat nausea during chemotherapy and stimulate weight gain. Sativex, a drug approved for treating pain and spasms in multiple sclerosis, contains an equal mix of THC and CBD. More recently, CBD oil has garnered attention for its potential benefits in alleviating certain symptoms associated with autism in children. Some parents and caregivers report that CBD may help reduce anxiety, improve sleep patterns, and alleviate sensory sensitivities of their children. While research is ongoing, these anecdotal accounts suggest that CBD oil could offer a promising avenue for supporting the well-being of autistic children.

Nevertheless, the legality of cannabis oil is intricate. In the UK, cannabidiol is legal, and hemp or CBD oil products are accessible in high-street stores and through online sellers, provided their THC content remains below 0.2 percent. According to David Nutt, a neuropsychopharmacologist at Imperial College London, "THC is not psychoactive at this level." However, in many other countries, CBD remains illegal. For example, in the USA, it falls under schedule 1 controlled substances and can only be distributed in states where cannabis use is sanctioned. Nonetheless, a recent assessment by the World Health Organization could potentially reshape perceptions of CBD, which was found to lack any potential for abuse or dependence while demonstrating its efficacy in treating epilepsy and other medical conditions, such as autism!

Although there is some scientific data suggesting that THC could be effective in controlling seizures, its psychoactive properties have shifted the spotlight toward cannabidiol, particularly for childhood epilepsies that do not respond to conventional treatments. Recent high-quality, randomized, placebo-controlled trials have provided evidence of CBD effectiveness in treating severe forms of epilepsy like Lennox-Gastaut and Dravet syndromes. While the exact mechanism of action remains unknown, it is believed to involve the inhibition of neuronal activity and the reduction of brain inflammation. However, when it comes to commercially sourced cannabis oils used for seizure control, the evidence is largely anecdotal, and the concentrations of CBD and THC can vary widely. A study by the UK Food Standard Authority (FSA) in 2022 further underscored the uncertainties surrounding these products.

The FSA study revealed that the concentration and composition of off-the-shelf remedies are often inaccurate. This inconsistency can result in incorrect dosages and, in some cases, consumers unwittingly purchasing ineffective or even harmful products. Although most of the sampled oils contained close to their labelled CBD content, two samples exceeded the declared CBD amount, while edibles displayed more variation. Beverages were found to contain less CBD than claimed, with one sample containing no CBD at all. The CBD levels in chocolate bars were near the labelled values, while gummies had only half the declared amount. Additionally, THC was detected in 87% of the samples analysed, with 40% of these exceeding the legal limit outlined in current Home Office guidelines. The study also examined levels of heavy metals and pesticides, detecting trace amounts in many samples, but not at concentrations posing health concerns.

So, while some anecdotal evidence suggests that CBD oils may help alleviate agitation, anxiety, or improve sleep in children with certain conditions, the ambiguity surrounding the sourcing of such medications and remedies, coupled with the challenges of accurately determining dosages when purchasing non-prescription CBD products, raises significant concerns. This underscores the need for comprehensive regulation and evaluation procedures. For me and Jen, after conducting research, the answer was clear: it wasn't worth the risk to administer a non-prescription CBD product to Rory. However, if clinically tested and evaluated CBD products become available through the NHS and prescription, it would certainly merit consideration for some.

Currently, the UK government's aim in reviewing medical cannabis is to assess the therapeutic potential of cannabis-based products in the initial phase of the review. Promising products may be recommended for further evaluation in the subsequent phase, conducted by the Advisory Council for the Misuse of Drugs, a government body with the authority to propose changes to the legal status of cannabis and cannabinoids for medical use. This process is expected to pave the way for more relaxed regulations on cannabis-based medicine research. Currently, cannabis remains categorized as Schedule 1, the most restrictive classification, alongside substances like LSD, with no recognized medicinal use. This paradox hinders research, preventing the demonstration of the medicinal value of cannabis and its derivatives. Moving cannabis to Schedule 2, alongside substances like morphine and diamorphine (heroin), would enable doctors to prescribe it when medically necessary.

The overarching concern is that without stringent regulation and standardized testing protocols, parents and caregivers remain uncertain about the purity, consistency, and safety of CBD treatments for their children. Furthermore, the potential presence of higher-than-advertised levels of THC in some products could inadvertently expose children to the psychoactive effects, in addition to potentially affecting sleep patterns, as THC affects sleep latency (onsets) and acts much like alcohol as a sedative, impacting REM sleep, which plays a crucial role in memory consolidation, emotional processing, brain development, and dreaming. Not only could we potentially be affecting our child's sleep, but regular or chronic users of cannabis oil that may have a higher than indicated level of THC could build up a tolerance to the sedating effects, resulting in the need for higher doses. Worse still, research suggests that stopping the remedy could cause horrific rebound effects of insomnia, essentially creating dependence if you wish to see the same benefits of an early onset of sleep in your child. CBD's effects on sleep, on the other hand, are perhaps more promising, but as yet not rigorously tested enough in neurotypical individuals, let alone developing neurodivergent brains. Therefore, the urgent need for comprehensive oversight, quality assurance measures, and standardized testing protocols cannot be overstated. This would provide parents with the confidence that the CBD products they use are safe and tailored to their children's unique needs.

As the discussion on cannabis evolves, with a shift from focusing solely on THC to exploring the influence of other cannabinoids like CBD on neural changes in both adolescents and adults, more information on consumable cannabis products is essential. This information is crucial in understanding their potential contribution to the development of psychiatric disorders and cognitive impairment in adulthood.

For now, the prudent course of action is to probably refrain from using non-prescription CBD products for children, given the uncertainties surrounding their composition and potency. The importance of rigorous regulation and evaluation cannot be overstated, especially when considering the well-being of young patients.

Vision & Glasses

Testing the eyesight of autistic children can be very challenging due to their unique characteristics. My goal is to share some valuable insights on how to approach eye examinations for our children based on my personal experiences, research, and information gathered from other parents and carers. However, I must admit that despite my efforts, I have not been able to take Rory to see an optometrist at an optician's office. I remain hopeful that with persistent attempts, like his dental visits, he might eventually be willing to undergo an eye examination. But, as of now, that possibility hasn't become a reality.

Understanding the signs, recommended assessments, and practical strategies, I again hope to empower parents and caregivers to support their child's visual health effectively.

Observing Potential Signs of Eyesight Difficulties:

Recognizing potential eyesight issues in autistic children requires a keen eye for subtle signs. Since these children may not always express their visual challenges verbally, it is essential to be attentive to behavioural cues. Some indicators that may suggest eyesight difficulties in autistic children include:

- *Frequent rubbing of eyes or squinting*
- *Holding objects unusually close to their face or at an odd angle*
- *Consistent difficulty with eye contact or focusing on people's faces.*
- *Avoiding activities that require visual tracking, such as reading or puzzles.*
- *Appearing disoriented or clumsy in their movements*

Seeking Professional Evaluation:

If you suspect that your autistic child is experiencing eyesight difficulties, consulting with an eye care professional is vital. Optometrists or ophthalmologists with experience in working with autistic children can perform comprehensive eye exams tailored to their unique needs.

Exams for Autistic Children:

Conducting eye exams for autistic children often requires adaptations to suit their sensory and communication preferences. Some tests that may be useful in evaluating their eyesight include:

Visual Acuity Test:

The optometrist will assess the child's ability to see letters, numbers, or pictures at various distances.

Eye Tracking and Teamwork:

Tests like the "Hirschberg Test" can help evaluate the child's ability to align their eyes and follow objects accurately.

Autorefractor:

This device measures the child's eye prescription objectively, reducing the need for verbal responses.

Teller Acuity Cards:

A preferred method for young or nonverbal children, this test uses visual reinforcement techniques to gauge their visual acuity.

Creating a Supportive Testing Environment:

Maintaining a supportive and accommodating environment during the eye exam is essential for a successful assessment. Provide your child with familiar comfort items, such as toys or blankets, to ease anxiety. Encourage the eye care professional to use visual aids, like picture charts or visual schedules, to facilitate communication.

Like all the challenges we face as parents and care givers Testing eyesight is no different for our children and requires patience, understanding, and specialized assessment techniques. By being attentive to potential signs, seeking professional evaluation, and ensuring a supportive testing environment, we can better understand and address visual challenges in these children.

Chapter XVII

Stimming

"Stimming is like turning down the radio when you think somethings burning. It's a way of turning off the other senses so you can make sure nothing is burning." - Lamar Hardwick

Though when most individuals think of stimming, they might initially associate it with autistic individuals, envisioning children who flap their hands or rock back and forth. However, the reality is that stimming is not exclusive to autism and is, in fact, a common behaviour across various neurotypes. Whenever I get anxious, usually while waiting for something imminent to happen, like seeing the dentist or receiving a test result, I begin to pace back and forth if I'm up and on my feet. Alternatively, if seated, I jiggle my leg and knee up and down in a repetitive manner. Likewise, if I'm annoyed and agitated, I tap my fingers and clench my jaw. I'm almost never aware I'm undertaking these actions unless they are pointed out to me. Chances are you have similar mannerisms - you might whistle unknowingly or draw little doodles while on the phone.

But I remember a time when I had no idea what the word autism was, let alone some of the characteristics associated with it like stimming. Yet, the sight of Rory giggling and flapping his hands was endearing and made his mother and me smile or laugh at this new mannerism, which started to appear around eighteen months to two years of age. This, as I was to later discover, was sometimes associated with autism.

But let's first explore some other examples of neurotypical individuals engaging in stimming in their everyday lives. People without any diagnosis may stim by biting their nails, twirling their hair absentmindedly, or pacing while talking on the phone. These actions provide sensory input and can be helpful for managing stress and anxiety, even for neurotypical individuals. For instance, someone might listen to music through headphones, use a fidget toy, or play with objects to relax and focus. Stimulating behaviours can be enjoyable ways to express oneself and find relief.

Stimming itself is short for self-stimulatory behaviour, also known as stereotypy and is characterised by actions that soothe or stimulate the senses. It can take various forms for everyone, and there is no right or wrong way to stim. Autistic individuals might use stimming to cope with anxiety or stress, but it can also be a positive and helpful activity for everyone.

So, while Rory does still flap, it's now with far less regularity than before. Instead, it's nearly always smiles, and laughter accompanied by high-pitched squeals of delight, bouncing, and jumping, which signal his happiness and enjoyment. The signs of his frustration have also changed. When he was younger and non-verbal, frustration almost always manifested in the form of dropping to the floor on his back and banging the rear of his head against the ground—a horrifying sight and sound to witness. It was several years before it transitioned to him biting his own fist, hitting himself or others nearby, or throwing his toys or electronics as his new way of venting frustration or anger. When it comes to frustration, Rory and I have recently spoken and have been working towards either crying or hugging, or that both are acceptable and normal.

Examples of stimming include harmless mannerisms like hand flapping, pacing, or rocking, as well as repetitive vocalizations or self-stimulatory behaviours such as staring at lights or spinning objects. Some stims serve a purpose, providing proprioceptive input or helping to calm an individual during anxious moments. While stimming can be beneficial, some forms may become harmful, like head-banging, biting oneself, or picking at the skin. It's important to recognize the potential risks and avoid engaging in harmful stims. Stimming has numerous advantages for autistic individuals and neurotypical people alike. It can diffuse difficult situations, provide an outlet for excess energy, improve focus, and reduce stress levels. Even successful athletes, like Serena Williams, who uses stimming techniques to get into the zone before big events.

So, despite the common misconception that only autistic individuals stim, neurotypical people also engage in stimming. They might tap their fingers, hum, or clench their fists in response to different situations. In situations where stimming may not be possible or appropriate, there are coping strategies to manage stress and anxiety. Deep breathing, shaking out tension, and visualizing a happy place are effective ways to ground oneself and find calm. For those who find stimming helpful, it's essential to embrace it and incorporate appropriate stims and sensory activities into daily routines. Being proactive about managing stimming urges and seeking therapeutic support, if necessary, can also be beneficial.

Understanding the various types of stimming is essential in comprehending how individuals with ASD interact with their environment. Some other types of stimming include:

- *Verbal and Auditory Stimming: Repetitive speech, covering or tapping of ears, snapping fingers, or making high-pitched noises.*
- *Visual Stimming: Staring blankly at objects, lining up toys, blinking repeatedly, or turning lights on and off.*
- *Tactile Stimming: Rubbing or scratching hands or objects, repetitive hand motions, and tapping fingers repeatedly.*
- *Vestibular Stimming: Rocking back and forth, twirling or spinning, jumping repeatedly, or hanging upside down.*
- *Olfactory or Taste Stimming: Smelling objects, tasting unusual things, or licking hands or objects.*

For individuals on the autism spectrum, stimming serves as a crucial means of coping with the challenges they face in their sensory-rich world. Autistic individuals often experience heightened sensitivity to sensory inputs, such as loud noises, bright lights, or crowded environments. These overwhelming stimuli can lead to anxiety, stress, and emotional distress. Engaging in stimming behaviours allows autistic individuals to self-regulate and manage their emotional and sensory experiences. Repetitive movements, vocalizations, or sensory-seeking activities can block out overwhelming inputs, offer a sense of predictability, and provide a soothing anchor in an otherwise chaotic environment. For some autistic individuals, stimming can also serve as a form of expression and communication. When words fail to convey their feelings or experiences adequately, stimming can become a non-verbal way of expressing joy, frustration, or excitement.

Understanding the distinction between ordinary stimming and autistic stimming is essential. Ordinary stimming, as seen in neurotypical individuals, is often limited in frequency and intensity. It occurs in response to specific situations and can usually be controlled or adjusted depending on the circumstances. On the other hand, autistic stimming tends to be more pervasive, repetitive, and less easily controllable. Autistic individuals may engage in stimming throughout the day, regardless of the situation, and might not even be aware of their own stimming behaviour. It is crucial to avoid stigmatizing or pathologizing stimming in any form, but recognizing the differences between ordinary and autistic stimming can help promote understanding and support for autistic individuals' unique needs.

While stimming is a beneficial and necessary coping mechanism for many autistic individuals, there are times when certain stims might be disruptive or harmful. In such cases, it is essential to provide appropriate support and alternatives. Parents, caregivers, and educators can play a vital role in helping autistic individuals manage stimming effectively. Here are some strategies to consider:

Creating Sensory-Friendly Environments:

Modify the individual's surroundings to reduce triggers and sensory overload. Provide a quiet space or offer noise-cancelling headphones in crowded or noisy settings.

Sensory Diets:

Introduce sensory diets, which are structured schedules of sensory activities that can help reduce the need for stimming. Sensory diets can include activities that offer sensory input and regulation.

Stress Reduction Techniques:

Teach stress reduction techniques, such as deep breathing exercises, progressive muscle relaxation, or using stress balls.

Occupational Therapy:

Seek the guidance of occupational therapists who specialise in autism to develop individualized strategies for managing stimming behaviours.

Medication (as needed):

For some individuals, medications may be prescribed to reduce anxiety and manage sensory overload, which can indirectly help in reducing stimming.

Encouraging Self-Expression: Create an environment where autistic individuals feel safe and encouraged to express their emotions and needs, whether through stimming or other means.

Remember, the primary focus should always be on the well-being and comfort of the individual. Reducing stress and anxiety through supportive measures can help promote positive outcomes and enable autistic individuals to thrive in their daily lives. Understanding stimming as a natural and common behaviour across all neurotypes fosters a culture of acceptance and inclusivity. Instead of perceiving stimming solely through the lens of autism, we should celebrate the diverse ways individuals engage with their surroundings and manage their emotions. By recognizing and appreciating the role stimming plays in an individual's life, we can better support those who might face challenges associated with sensory processing and create an environment where everyone feels valued and understood. Promoting neurodiversity not only enriches the lives of neurodivergent individuals but also enhances our collective understanding of the human experience. Embracing stimming as a normal aspect of human behaviour empowers individuals to embrace their unique selves, promoting empathy and compassion in society.

So, stimming is a natural and common behaviour for individuals of all neurotypes. It serves various purposes, from managing emotions to providing sensory relief. If stimming is not harmful to oneself or others, it should be accepted and embraced. If anyone is concerned about their stimming behaviour, seeking professional help can provide valuable support and understanding. It's also worth noting that certain stims may intensify over time or may even disappear and be replaced by a new stim, as our children adapt, grow, and mitigate the challenges of the world.

Chapter XVIII

A Families Best Friend

"A dog is the only thing on earth that loves you more than you love yourself" – Josh Billings

My wife Jennifer, once made a comment shortly after we got our second puppy: *"It's like you prefer dogs more than people."* This statement is almost correct because it's all animals in general that I prefer to people, but dogs do tend to take greater preference.

Before I undertook my science degree, I pursued a diploma in canine psychology and behaviour. Although we are entirely different species, we have co-evolved closely, and more so than any other animal. It's with a sense of irony that our beloved family pets share many similarities with our autistic children. Their brains are wired in a manner entirely distinct from our own, to the extent that both parties essentially communicate in different languages, neither fully comprehending the other's. This difference, much like the behaviour of our children, may occasionally prove frustrating or even vexing to us.

For example, our dog is happily resting by our side when suddenly they jump up, ears pricked back, hackles raised along the spine, and they erupt into incessant barking due to a sound we may not have noticed. Yes, it's the sound of a potential predator and threat—it is the postman or mail carrier. Owners will often tell the pet to be quiet and may raise their voice and change tone to make a point. But to a dog, that raised voice and change in tone just says, *'Yes, you hear it too, master. My master is making his barking sound too. Let's continue to scare off this threat together.'*

The owner will often then get annoyed with the barking and continue to tell the dog to shut up, which again just reinforces the undesired behaviour. Or worse, the dog gets scolded and sent to its bed, and the dog is now completely at a loss as to what just happened. Because in their mind, they were doing what they always do when the mail is delivered—barking along with their human. It's a complete miscommunication on both the dog and the human's part, and the dog is likely to continue this undesired behaviour, much like a child would, unless the adult/human changes their behaviour first.

As mentioned before, you need to look at not just the subject but also the environment during undesired behaviour and see what's different and how we can change this, as well as how I can change my approach and communication to a form that might be understood by my child or, in this instance, my pet. The answer for the dog is simple: break the cycle of barking by not raising your voice and instead have a treat ready to distract the dog when they hear the mail carrier.

Eventually, the dog will stop barking, as it doesn't seem to bother you, and in fact, you are so content with the noise that you seem to give out food freely. Gradually replace treats with a pat or stroke in a relaxed manner, and the dog and you will soon be at ease during mail delivery time. The most important lesson here is that some of our behaviour and communication they understand, and some they don't. But they won't do anything about it because a dog loves you more than they love themselves. As humans, we sometimes don't understand this unconditional love, but the dog loves you unconditionally. If you do something they consider odd, they just consider it something you do and won't judge you, we as parents should embrace these oddities or differences in our own children and like our dog, just accept the differences.

According to my parents, my first pet was a cat called Midnight. Though I have no recollection of this feline friend, I'm told by my parents that it was more like a dog in nature. It would run after the family car when I was a baby and jump through the window to snuggle next to me. Unfortunately, as is so often the case living in a suburban area, Midnight came to an untimely end due to a road accident. My earliest memory of any pet was that of Jet, who was, as the name suggests, another cat that was jet black in appearance.

I remember that she had kittens when I must have been around eighteen months to two years of age. I also recall losing at least one kitten during birth and one of my parents trying to revive it. This was my first memorable encounter with death and confusion about the subject.

A few weeks later, the kittens had grown, and for some reason, I must have confused bats and cats, as I had the idea that these creatures should be able to fly. So, perhaps showing an early aptitude for science and physics in particular, I proceeded to drop some kittens over the third-floor apartment balcony. Thankfully and as we all know, cats, even little ones, have a reflex that allows them to land on their feet. I'm happy to report that all the kittens that experienced this skydiving adventure survived. My grandmother took two and named them Tom and Ollie, and they lived to a ripe old age.

When I was five years old, we moved to the same grandparents' spacious home, which was fantastic because I now had a 100ft garden that backed onto a wooded country park. There were streams, ponds, and an abundance of wildlife. This period in my life unquestionably contributed to my love of animals and the natural world in general. My grandparents were animal lovers, and we always had at least four or more dogs, two cats, and at times, we also had chickens, rabbits, guinea pigs, exotic birds (my favourite being an African Grey called Monty, who mimicked my mother's bad language at untimely moments), as well as various tropical and cold-water fish and numerous rodents. It's safe to say that my time in that household nurtured my love for all living creatures. My grandfather

184

and father would often take me on walks and teach me about hedgerow foods and herbs. Everyone encouraged my curiosity about the living world, so it wasn't surprising that I would find and keep frogs, toads, newts, and even a grass snake that one of the cats brought home, which happened to be one of the kittens I had dropped over the balcony years before. But of all the animals, the ones I had the most interaction with were the dogs, and they were always of different breeds. My favourites were two toy poodles named Winston and Trudy. Growing up around dogs of different breeds as a child allowed me to become attuned to their quirks and behaviours.

Trudy, in particular, was mischievous and became my personal favourite when I was five years old. She joined me on adventures in the garden and around the house, and she was certainly the alpha of the pack for some time. Trudy would follow me like a mother hen wherever I went, which gave me reassurance in the darker and foreboding parts of the garden and the country park. I would often lift the chain-link fence that separated the bottom of the garden from the park, and we would go off on adventures together without telling anyone in the household.

Later in my childhood, after my parents and I moved out and got our own dog, a Labrador cross Border Collie puppy named Bo-Bo, who was initially intended to be my brother's pet. During the transition period of settling into a new life with us, Bo-Bo was restless and confused and would whine during the night. To comfort her, I brought my bedding down from my bedroom and slept on the kitchen floor. Since I was the older child and more independent, I often walked Bo-Bo myself, and a bond was quickly formed between us. Since Bo-Bo, all my dogs, except for one rescue dog, have been of the same mixed breed. Nowadays, they are called Boradors, which to me sounds like a regional province or land, alongside Mordor and Gondor from the Lord of the Rings novels. Due to my continued adventurous immersion with nature during my transition from child to teenager, Bo-Bo became my best friend and joined me on all my treks through woodlands. I would also sit and read under a tree by my favourite pond in the country park, often referred to as "The Manor" by locals it was the same park I frequented as a child. Bo-Bo was my most consistent friend and lived a good number of years before passing away around the age of fifteen.

My son was born and raised alongside our recently deceased dog, Poppy. She was a fantastic companion to me and literally followed me everywhere around the home. As she was the most well-behaved of my now four dogs, she would also accompany me to friends and family homes while the younger dogs stayed at home. It wasn't until Rory came to live with Jennifer and I permanently in 2017 that he started inquiring more frequently about Poppy. At the time, Poppy had stayed behind with my ex-wife in the family home, as we were not allowed to have pets in our apartment. It was a surprise to realize that Rory was now frequently asking about the dog, which meant that he not only acknowledged her but also missed her presence and company. Looking back at old photos and videos, I realized how much Poppy was also Rory's shadow at times. During mealtimes, Rory would place unwanted food under the table which would often find its way to Poppy, and as Rory grew older, she would lick his face to remove food and sauces. Rory learned to throw a ball before he learned to walk, and he was always delighted to see his furry companion retrieve the ball for him.

Even after moving back to the family home with the children in 2018, one of my old neighbours approached me and mentioned how they enjoyed watching Rory and Poppy bouncing on the garden trampoline. Rory would throw the ball for his canine friend, and she would be catapulted in the air every second or so upon returning the ball to Rory's feet.

While I am a strong advocate for people owning dogs and the benefits they can bring as domesticated animals, especially as assistance dogs that enable their owners' independence or help with everyday tasks, there are many other advantages and disadvantages as well. Owning a dog can provide companionship, reduce stress, and blood pressure, improve sociability, and contribute to overall well-being and health. One study found that children in homes with pets, who are involved in their care, showed signs of empathy sooner or developed it earlier. Another study indicated a reduced risk of developing respiratory and ear infections, gastroenteritis, and some allergies. Additionally, walking and interacting with a dog can provide exercise, leading to healthier children and higher school attendance. Another pilot study discovered that children aged five to eight from pet-owning families achieved two to three extra weeks of school attendance.

I recall watching a made-for-TV movie in 2006, titled "After Thomas" that emotionally impacted me at the time because it was about a young boy who was disconnected from the world around him. Yet when a puppy came into his life, things changed. Whether that be due to the dog's arrival or the boy learning to find coping mechanisms as he developed and grew older, we'll never truly be able to tell from a ninety-minute movie. But I'd like to think that, like Rory's interaction with Poppy, any dog can positively benefit an individual and/or a family unit.

Unfortunately, during the movie, Thomas ages and sadly passes. This is a common experience all pet owners, particularly dog owners, must prepare for, and that time came for our own furry family member recently. But even with the passing of Poppy, it gave us the opportunity to discuss her death with Rory.

We engaged in a conversation about the inevitability of death for all living things and how that reality feels in the present. We offered reassurance to him, explaining that it's acceptable to feel sadness in such situations because it's a testament to the love and companionship we enjoyed with the departed. We emphasized that this emotional experience signifies the depth of our connections, something we cherish and wish to preserve.

Bringing Poppy back home, we allowed everyone to bid their farewells. However, both Rory and Rose consciously opted to retain their memories of Poppy as she was. Though this choice likely stemmed from a desire to avoid the sight of their tearful and emotional father, overcome with grief, and attempting to bury Poppy in the front yard. I can confirm that passersby quickly stopped and returned the way they came upon encountering this poignant scene: a visibly emotional man, clutching a shovel, standing beside a shallow grave with Poppy's body wrapped in a blanket which to them must have resembled a small child. It's a wonder I didn't attract the attention of the local authorities with my display of emotions and the improvised burial arrangement.

During the research phase for this book, I came across the movie mentioned, "After Thomas," and discovered that it was based on the lives of a real autistic family, the Gardners, and their son, Dale. If you're interested, you can read about their story in Nuala Gardner's 2008 book, 'A Friend Like Henry'

Advantages of Dog Ownership-

Emotional Support:

One of the primary benefits of getting a dog for an autistic child is emotional support. Many autistic children struggle with social interactions and may have difficulty expressing themselves or understanding the emotions of others. However, dogs can provide a source of unconditional love and support, which can help children feel more secure and connected to the world around them.

Increased Social Interaction:

Some autistic children may have difficulty interacting with others, but dogs can provide a bridge to social interaction. For example, a dog can be a conversation starter, as children can talk about their dog with others and share stories about their pet. Additionally, caring for a dog can provide opportunities for social interaction, such as taking the dog for walks or going to dog parks, which can help autistic children develop social skills and make friends.

Physical Activity:

Any children that struggle with physical activity, which could lead to health problems such as obesity and cardiovascular disease. May benefit having a dog can provide a source of motivation for physical activity, as children can take the dog for walks or play with them in the yard. This can help improve the overall physical health of autistic children and reduce the risk of health problems associated with a sedentary lifestyle.

Reduced Anxiety:

Dogs can provide a source of comfort and calm for all neurotypes, which can help reduce anxiety and stress. For example, petting a dog can have a calming effect and release endorphins, which may improve mood and reduce anxiety. Additionally, dogs can provide a sense of security, as some autistic children may feel anxious in unfamiliar environments or situations.

Improved Communication:

Dogs can provide a way for autistic children to practice communication skills. For example, children may learn to give commands to their dog and communicate with others about their pet. Additionally, dogs may provide a source of motivation for communication, as children may be more willing to talk to others about their dog than other topics. Much like the aforementioned movie "After Thomas"

Responsibility and Independence:

Caring for a dog can provide opportunities for children to develop responsibility and independence. For example, children may learn to feed and care for their dog, which can help them develop a sense of responsibility and self-sufficiency. Additionally, caring for a dog can provide a sense of accomplishment and help children develop a sense of pride in their ability to care for another living creature.

Sensory Stimulation:

Children with sensory processing difficulties may struggle with certain types of sensory input. However, dogs may provide a source of sensory stimulation that is soothing and calming for autistic children. For example, petting a dog can provide tactile stimulation, while the sound of a dog's breathing can provide auditory stimulation. Additionally, interacting with a dog can provide opportunities for sensory integration and modulation, which can help improve overall sensory processing abilities.

Improved Executive Functioning:

Our children may struggle with executive functioning, which can make it challenging to complete tasks and manage daily routines. However, caring for a dog can help improve executive functioning in several ways. For example, having a dog can provide a structured routine, such as feeding and walking times, which can help children with ASC learn to manage their time and develop organizational skills.

Increased Empathy:

Empathy is the ability to understand and share the feelings of others. Some autistic children may struggle with empathy but caring for a dog may provide additional opportunities to develop this important social skill. For example, children may learn to recognize when their dog is happy, sad, or in need of attention, which can help them develop a better understanding of the emotions of others.

Disadvantages of Dog Ownership:

Cost:

One of the primary disadvantages of getting a dog for anyone is the cost. Dogs require food, veterinary care, and other supplies, which can be expensive. Additionally, unexpected veterinary expenses can arise, such as emergency care or surgeries, which can add to the cost of owning a dog.

Time Commitment:

Caring for a dog requires a significant time commitment, which may be challenging for some families. For example, dogs need to be fed, exercised, and groomed regularly, which can be time-consuming. Additionally, families may need to adjust their schedules to accommodate the needs of their dog, which may be difficult for families with busy schedules or limited resources.

Allergies:

Some children may have allergies to dogs, which can make it difficult to own a dog. Allergies can cause symptoms such as sneezing, itching, and respiratory problems, which can be disruptive to daily life. Additionally, families may need to take special precautions to reduce allergens in the home, such as vacuuming regularly or using air filters.

Safety Concerns:

Dogs may also pose safety concerns for autistic children, particularly if the child is unable to communicate effectively or if the dog is not trained properly. For example, a dog may become aggressive if provoked or may bite if the child is not handling the dog properly.

Additionally, some dogs may have a high prey drive, which can be dangerous for small children.

Hygiene:

Dogs and especially puppies can be messy and may require regular grooming to maintain hygiene. For example, dogs may shed, drool, or track in dirt and mud, which can be challenging for families to manage. Additionally, families may need to clean up after their dog, such as picking up waste in the yard or cleaning up accidents in the house.

Training:

Training a dog can be challenging, particularly if the dog is a puppy or has behavioural issues. Families may need to invest time and resources in training their dog, such as attending obedience classes or working with a professional trainer. Additionally, families may need to be patient and consistent in their training efforts, which can be difficult for some families.

These are the most obvious advantages and disadvantages to getting a dog for an autistic child like Rory. While dogs can provide emotional support, increased social interaction, and physical activity, they can also be costly, time-consuming, and pose safety concerns. Families should carefully consider the potential benefits and drawbacks of getting a dog for their autistic child before making a decision that affects two lives. Additionally, when it comes to sharing a home with an autistic child, selecting a breed of dog with an easy temperament is important. Considering that an autistic child may exhibit challenging behaviours, such as hitting or pulling on the dog, it is crucial to choose a breed that can thrive in a family environment. Some breeds are more likely than others to tolerate and benefit from the behaviours of autistic children. Selecting the right breed of dog for a child with autism can be a difficult decision, as different breeds have different temperaments, energy levels, and requirements. Some breeds are better suited to living with children with autism due to their calm and friendly personalities, while others may not be as well-suited. Here are some of the best dog breeds for children with autism and the reasons why they are a good fit-

Golden Retriever:

Golden Retrievers are one of the most popular breeds for families with children with autism. They are known for their friendly and gentle nature and are very social, making them great companions for children with autism. They are also highly trainable, making them well-suited for therapy and service work. Golden Retrievers are also very patient and tolerant, which is important when living with children with autism who may have sensory processing issues or difficulty controlling their movements. Additionally, they have a high energy level and love to play, which can provide children with autism with the opportunity for physical activity and sensory stimulation.

Labrador Retriever:

Labrador Retrievers are another popular breed for families with children with autism. They are known for their friendly and outgoing personalities and are highly trainable, making them well-suited for service work. They are also great with children and are very patient, which is important when living with children with autism who may have difficulty controlling their movements or understanding social cues. Labrador Retrievers are also very active and love to play, which can provide children with autism with the opportunity for physical activity and sensory stimulation. Additionally, they are very loyal and form strong bonds with their families, which can provide emotional support and companionship for children with autism.

Poodle:

Poodles are a great choice for families with children with allergies, as they have a hypoallergenic coat that does not shed. They are also highly intelligent and trainable, making them well-suited for service work and therapy. Poodles are also very loyal and affectionate, making them great companions for children with autism. They are also very adaptable and can adjust to different environments and living situations, which can be helpful for families with children with autism who may have difficulty with change.

Cavalier King Charles Spaniel:

Cavalier King Charles Spaniels are known for their friendly and affectionate personalities and are great companions for children with autism. They are also very social and enjoy being around people, which can provide children with autism with opportunities for social interaction and companionship. Cavalier King Charles Spaniels are also very adaptable and can adjust to different environments and living situations, which can be helpful for families with children with autism who may have difficulty with change. Additionally, they are a smaller breed, making them well-suited for families who live in apartments or smaller homes.

Border Collie:

Border Collies are known for their high energy level and intelligence, making them well-suited for families with children with autism who need a lot of physical activity and mental stimulation.

They are also highly trainable and are often used for service work and therapy. Border Collies are also very loyal and affectionate and form strong bonds with their families. They are also very patient and tolerant, which is important when living with children with autism who may have sensory processing issues or difficulty controlling their movements.

Bernese Mountain Dog:

Bernese Mountain Dogs are known for their gentle and friendly nature and are great companions for children with autism. They are also very patient and tolerant, which is important when living with children with autism who may have sensory processing issues or difficulty controlling their movements. Bernese Mountain Dogs are also very loyal and form strong bonds with their families. They are also very adaptable and can adjust to different environments and living situations, which can be helpful for families with children with autism who may have difficulty with change. Additionally, Bernese Mountain Dogs are a larger breed, which can provide a sense of security and comfort for children with autism. They also have a thick, soft coat, which can provide sensory stimulation and comfort for children who may benefit from tactile input.

Beagle:

Beagles are known for their friendly and playful personalities and are great companions for children with autism. They are also highly adaptable and can adjust to different environments and living situations, which can be helpful for families with children with autism who may have difficulty with change. Beagles are also very patient and tolerant, which is important when living with children with autism who may have sensory processing issues or difficulty controlling their movements. Additionally, they have a high energy level and love to play, which can provide children with autism with the opportunity for physical activity and sensory stimulation.

It is important to note that while these breeds may be well-suited for living with children with autism, every dog is an individual with their own personality and behaviour. It is important to spend time with the dog or puppy and assess their compatibility with the child before making a final decision. Additionally, consulting with a professional dog trainer or behaviourist can be helpful in selecting the right breed and individual dog for a child with autism. Dogs, as we know, evolved from a now-extinct species of wolf, no longer present in its original form due to selective breeding. Dogs have been bred to exhibit the qualities humans find most desirable and useful when living alongside us. While each breed may look different, it's important to consider their wolf ancestry. Sometimes, an old wolf trait or characteristic may drive a dog to inflict harm on a human or even kill. However, it's worth noting that out of the UKs sixteen million dogs, only a very small fraction of dangerous behaviour towards humans is ever reported. In comparison, we, the so-called socialized apes, commit more atrocities and killings among ourselves on a daily basis than any dog does. Dogs will generally do everything they can to keep their family safe if someone tries to harm you or even if you try to harm yourself. They truly are human's best friend.

As of 2023, our canine companions remain at a count of four. Among them are three Border Collie x Labradors, ranging in age from five to seven years old. Following Poppy's departure, there's a noticeable gap within our family. Our most recent inclusion is a seven-month-old Belgian Malinois x German Shepherd hybrid. I must emphasize that this particular breed or crossbreed is not one I would recommend for individuals who are inexperienced or new to dog ownership.

Acknowledgements

I would like to extend my heartfelt gratitude to the incredible parents, carers, and educators whom I've had the privilege to meet over the years. Whether we connected at parenting clubs, online forum groups, or academic settings like schools, your unwavering dedication and willingness to share your experiences and knowledge about the diverse challenges of autism have been invaluable. Your insights have been as inspiring as the condition itself is complex.

My best friend Bryan, whose wise and balanced advice has been a constant source of support, even though he and his family are no longer living close by. He has played a crucial role in inspiring me to write a book for fathers and explore the challenges we face. Without his initial input, my book might not have encompassed important subjects like my personal struggles with depression and thoughts of suicide.

To my parents, even though we may have had our differences over the years, your unwavering love and concern for my well-being and education have been the cornerstone of my ability to support and care for my own young family. Your lifelong support has given me the strength to follow a similar path with my children in that family comes first over money and material wealth.

I would also like to express my appreciation to my aunts and uncles, whose collective wisdom and balanced guidance were instrumental during my childhood. A special thank you goes to my auntie Jackie, who played the role of a caring big sister whenever I needed guidance as a young teenager.

My gratitude extends to my grandparents, who took an active interest in my upbringing and early fascination with the natural world. Their encouragement led me to pursue an environmental science degree and shaped my love for the great outdoors.

This book is dedicated to two of the most influential figures in my life. First, my great grandmother Louisa Rose, whose influence, even in her absence of twenty years, continues to guide me. Her lessons in independence, standing up for beliefs, and showing compassion for others resonate with me to this day.

To my beloved son, Rory, you are the most influential person in my life. Your mischievous and cheeky nature have taught me valuable lessons about myself, the human condition, and the beauty of being a unique individual and not worrying what others think.

To my wonderful stepchildren, Apollo, George, and Emily, I am incredibly grateful and touched by your acceptance and understanding as I became a part of your lives. Your warmth and support during my darkest hours have been a guiding light, and I cherish the love and care you've shown me.

Furthermore, I want to express my deepest appreciation for the way you welcomed my own children into our home with open hearts and open arms. Your kindness and inclusivity have created a loving and nurturing family environment that means the world to me.

Special thanks are due to my ex-wife, Phoebe, for giving me the gift of two amazingly different and diverse children.

Lastly, my deepest appreciation goes to my wife, Jennifer. Your love, encouragement, empathy, and unwavering support fuel my every endeavour. You are my Mary Poppins, "Practically Perfect in every way," and I couldn't imagine this journey without you by my side. Thank you for making every day extraordinary.

With sincere gratitude,

Matt

About the Author

Matthew resides in Essex, England, where he shares his home with his two children, Rose and Rory, and second wife, Jennifer. Their lively household is also home to four dogs, two cats, chicken's honeybees, and exotic birds. With a lifelong passion for animals, wildlife, and the wonders of nature, Matthew's love for the environment eventually led him to pursue a degree in environmental science through the Open University.

A strong advocate of climate change awareness, wildlife conservation, and education, Matthew is deeply committed to preserving natural biodiversity and promoting acceptance of human cultural, ethnic, and neurological diversity. His dedication to understanding and supporting those with unique differences and challenges is an integral part of his journey.

Currently, Matthew is embarking on a new chapter in his life as he undertakes the path to obtain his qualified teacher status. His aspiration is to make a meaningful difference as an educator in a Special Needs School, continuing to learn and grow alongside those he has the privilege to teach and learn from.

Beyond his academic pursuits. Together with his son Rory, they are embarking on their second book chronicling their journey through Rory's teenage years and Matthew's middle age. This heartfelt project will hope to capture their shared experiences, challenges, and growth, emphasizing the enduring bond between father and son.

Through this book and in life Matthew hopes to inspire others to appreciate the beauty of the natural world, embrace diversity, and foster a greater sense of compassion for all living things. His mission is to create a positive impact on both the environment and the lives of those around him, making the world a better place for future generations.

Printed in Great Britain
by Amazon

28959478R00116